What caregivers and writers say about *Musical Morphine*

I WAS CAPTURED from the first moment I started reading Robin Gaiser's *Musical Morphine: Transforming Pain One Note at a Time*. It tells with amazing openness about the lessons she learned, the joys and sorrows given and received working with the ill and dying. As a hospice nurse of many years, I felt this could have been my story. —Kathleen Jablonski, RN, Hospice, retired

MUSICAL MORPHINE TAKES the reader on a positive and sometimes very emotional journey of dedication, hope, and warmth as Robin Gaiser tells the stories of the lives that she has touched as a musician, healer, and loving human being. She embraces the challenges of her patients' pain and despair and demonstrates how her music nurtures the sick and infirm in beautiful, positive ways on their personal transitional journeys. A must read.

—Nick Jacobs, B.S., M.Ed., MPM, FACHE
Chairman, Clinical and Translational Genome Research Institute
Fort Myers, Florida

AS MUCH A story about finding your own path as it is story of music's balm for the sick and dying, *Musical Morphine* offers insight into healthcare that places care of the soul at its center. A moving, inspiring, and hope-giving book for individuals and hospital administrators alike. May a therapeutic musician be in the room with me when I go. —Laura Hope-Gill
Director, Thomas Wolfe Center for Narrative
Narrative Medicine Program, Lenoir-Rhyne University

THIS BOOK BEAUTIFULLY captures and reveals the many mysteries and miracles that occur regularly in the work of any therapeutic musician, and how our training through the Music for Healing and Transition Program guides us in navigating the sometimes murky waters of therapeutic music. I found myself nodding in agreement, or smiling, laughing, or crying in sympathy, and seeing myself and my patients in almost every story. *Been there! Done that!* Yes, but I never could have expressed it so masterfully.

Thank you, Robin. *Musical Morphine* is not just your story, but the story of therapeutic music in America, told in a readable, entertaining, and meaningful way. This book will help anyone ... musician, a health care professional, or a hospital administrator, understand the importance of therapeutic music in health care today, particularly for those who are critically ill or dying. —Earl Fowler, J.D., CMP
Chief District Court Judge, retired

MUSICAL MORPHINE INTERTWINES one woman's journey through grief with her ability to move through that same experience with others, assisted by a handful of instruments and her mastery of lyric, melody and rhythm. Music, through its many layers and forms, is intrinsically built to accompany end-of-life experiences and all the emotions that arise on that path. There is such a need. So, come on in, there's plenty of room. And, as you will learn as you turn these pages, results can be simply life-changing. —Lara McKinnis, M.S., MT-BC

LOVELY AND MOVING! [Gaiser] writes with reverence and restraint, letting the stories naturally unfold. The writing has a wonderful, quiet rhythm.
—Laurel Hunt, pet therapy volunteer, Mission Health System, Asheville, NC
author, *Pawprints: Reflections on Loving and Losing a Canine Companion*

AS A PHYSICIAN, I often see patients struggle through illness and suffer the limits of medical interventions. The[se] stories reveal the art in healing and sometimes, despite our best efforts, the art in dying. As a healthcare music practitioner, Gaiser offers not only joy to the listener but an anesthetic for the patient.

I recently experienced the death of a dear friend whose passing was made easier through the melodies of a harpist. Her breathing gently slowed to the peaceful rhythm of the music as she died surrounded by friends, family, and the sounds that had sustained her throughout her life. In this book, Robin shares her experiences that illustrate the profound effect that music can have in awakening the joy in patients' hearts, healing broken relationships in families, and liberating dying souls with grace. —Susan Mims, M.D., M.P.H., FAAP
Mission Health System

AS A HOSPICE physician who spends time at the bedsides of the dying, I'm interested in the stories of other professionals who do similar work: how they came to be there, why they stayed. Robin Gaiser offers just such a story about her experience as a certified music practitioner for people who are chronically or terminally ill, full of her own motivations, her musical talents, and the well-described lives and deaths of the people she served. You'll learn about the transformations that occur, not just in the recipients of her music, but in the giver as well. That she was able to bring these skills to her dying parents, described in the stories that open and close the book, make the reading experience even more moving. Once you read what music can do when you're ill, you'll want to have someone like Robin at your bedside. —Claire Hicks, M.D.
Hospice and Palliative Care physician, Asheville, NC

"There is a deep and mysterious paradox here, for while such music makes one experience pain and grief more intensely, it brings solace and consolation at the same time. " — Oliver Sacks, *Musicophilia*

THIS IS ONE of the wise quotes Robin Gaiser has selected to punctuate her powerful narrative about relationships with family, friendship, pain, joy, and love through the gift of music. The reader is privy to sacred moments with people at their most vulnerable through Gaiser's generous story-telling.

In addition to music, Gaiser brings a religious literacy and sensitivity, knowing that human beings have such complicated relationships with the spiritual traditions of their childhood, and sometimes what is needed is a song that can touch that part. Other times what is needed is a German drinking song or "Let Me Call You Sweetheart." *Musical Morphine* sings of courage, encounter, and peace.

—Katharine R. Meacham, Ph.D.
Professor of Philosophy and Religion, Mars Hill University
Adjunct Professor, Dept. of Social Medicine, UNC SOMS-Asheville, NC

LOVELY MOVING STORIES ... Chill-bump prose.

—Tommy Hays, author, *The Pleasure Was Mine*
Director, Great Smokies Writing Program, UNC Asheville

IN *MUSICAL MORPHINE*, Robin Gaiser opens a fascinating window into the world of a Certified Music Practitioner by tracing her initial inklings about the field, through the life-developments that opened the practice to her, to joining healing teams. But the deeper import of this highly readable volume is how the specific musical gifts of one person contribute to others as they face the inevitable limits of their finitude ...

Gaiser is honest about occasional misjudgments, but she always [seeks] the way music can bring wholeness. Most of the people to whom she ministered with her music did not get "better"; in fact, most of them died. But with the power of music, their living until their end was indeed better. And in the process of reading this book, a lot is learned about living and dying well. — D. Cameron Murchison
Professor of Ministry, emeritus, Columbia Theological Seminary
Transitional Pastoral Associate, Grace Covenant Presbyterian Church, Asheville, NC

I GOT SO emotionally involved, [despite] not knowing much about the people described. But ... providing background on dying folks' need for resolution and the lyrics to those old hymns and songs is really powerful.

—Dwight Martin, M.F.A. student, Queens University, Charlotte, NC

NOTHING BEATS READING this book through in its entirety. I laughed and cried, got angry, and rejoiced as I journeyed along. The stories of each patient touched my heart ... and I wanted to hear more, to meet one more patient, to hear one more song.

I would recommend this book to any and all who connect with the elderly, the sick and the dying. Robin Gaiser gives a beautiful example of each patient's condition and the spirit she brought to each one, through music, through settling herself, showing her compassion, understanding, weakness and strength.

Gaiser writes, "While others give money, feed the hungry ... I make music. Not simply because I can, because it's what I do, but because music reaches into a restless, hungry place within me ...."

I found myself crying out, "Yes, that's it!"   —Donna Castaner, CMP student

IN *MUSICAL MORPHINE*, Gaiser chronicles her vocational journey of becoming a Certified Musical Practitioner. The individual stories that comprise this collection combine to provide the reader with insight into Gaiser's personal and professional development. The author brings the fullness of her own life experience to play as she reaches out to those with critical needs, providing distraction, healing, comfort, and peace. Gaiser's personal struggles are beautifully woven into each recounted vignette demonstrating that the transformational gift of music so freely shared with her patients, in the end becomes the very prescription that sustains and empowers her work.   —William J. Jones, DMA
Director, Music Ministries
Grace Covenant Presbyterian Church

IP

Pisgah Press was established in 2011 to publish and promote works of quality offering original ideas and insight into the human condition and the world around us.

Printed in the United States of America

Published by Pisgah Press, LLC
PO Box 1427, Candler, NC 28715
www.pisgahpress.com

Book design: A. D. Reed, MyOwnEditor.com
Cover design and photo by Laurie McCarriar, www.artistgeek.com
Back cover photo by Bonnie Cooper, www.bonniecooperphotography.com

"Excerpt" from the book *BEING MORTAL: Medicine and What Matters in the End* by Atul Gawande. Copyright © 2014 by Atul Gawande. Used by permission of Henry Holt and Company, LLC. All rights reserved.

Library of Congress Cataloging-in-Publication Data
Gaiser, Robin Russell
Musical Morphine/Robin Gaiser, CMP

Library of Congress Control Number: 2016939202

ISBN-13: 978-1942016175
ISBN-10: 1942016174
Philosophy / Ethics & Moral philosophy

First Printing
June 2016

Musical MORPHINE

Transforming Pain One Note at a Time

Robin Russell Gaiser, CMP

Disclaimer

This book is not an instruction manual. As a memoir it is my unique experience, not the story of one institution, one organization or one profession, although specific references are made to them for the sake of clarity.

The differences between Music Therapists and Music Practitioners merit explanation. I am not a music therapist; rather, I am a therapeutic musician, known as a Certified Music Practitioner (CMP). Music therapists obtain at least one college degree in Music Therapy; once licensed, they provide patients with a prescribed clinical application of musical activities aimed at improving cognitive, physical, psychological, or social functioning. Their work is focused on achieving a specific therapeutic goal.

A CMP, who obtains certification through Music for Healing and Transition, Inc., spends two to three years in intensive training and practicum experience. Music is offered not as a prescriptive application but, rather, to create an environment at the bedside (or chair-side) of the critically and chronically ill, the elderly, and the dying in which the natural resources of patients' bodies and minds—to calm anxiety, reduce cardio stress, respond to medication, or simply rest—can come into play. Live, usually acoustic, music is not seen as curative (nor is it "entertainment"); it is, however, therapeutic.

Many of the musical activities of Music Therapists and Music Practitioners overlap. Both professions sponsor ongoing research studying the far-reaching effects of music on the groups they serve in hopes of increasing the presence of music in medical settings.

The reader is advised to seek professional guidance when applying any of the practices and policies referred to in *Musical Morphine*. For a partial listing of recommended resources, visit www.robingaiser.com/resources. The reader may contact me for more information via my website, Facebook page, or at robingaiser@gmail.com.

Foreword

Death. Life-limiting illness. Subjects that both intrigue and frighten.

How did America become such a death-defying culture? Our ancestors were well acquainted with the reality of dying. Learned people spent entire careers studying and explaining it. We all have a departure date, yet we behave as if it were optional.

In Robin Russell Gaiser's book, we will witness that decline and death are part of life, a continuum that cannot be explained in a linear Cartesian fashion, cannot be broken, but can be accepted as an inseparable link in a never-ending cycle. The song "Will the Circle Be Unbroken" comes to mind, posing the question whether death breaks the circle of life; the lyrics answer with a resounding "No!" The circle continues despite the physical disappearance of one of its links.

I met Robin at a musical jam session in my own home. I was a beginning fiddle student who had learned recently that I might have a serious illness. To my relief, surgery for my condition brought forth benign results, but the experience forced me to examine what, otherwise, I might have missed: music rose to the top of the list.

During high school in Oneida, N.Y., I spent my time practicing to be a virtuoso clarinetist and working as a nurses' aide in the local hospital. When a college decision had to be made, I chose music education over nursing and headed off to Mount Union College. There, in addition to clarinet, I was required to excel at playing the piano. That did not happen, so I transferred to Syracuse University's School of Nursing. Later I obtained a Nurse Practitioner certificate, followed by a Masters in Science, and for twenty-four years I worked as a Family Nurse Practitioner in primary care.

I also raised a family, and music sat on the back burner, while I felt like a heart-sick lover waiting for the chance to dive into making music again. Just when I began the fiddle lessons and met Robin, we both discovered the Music for Healing and Transition Program, Inc., which trained musicians to become Certified Music Practitioners. We applied, were accepted, and took courses; then, still together, we fulfilled our internship at Mountain Valley Hospice in Gloversville, N.Y. As CMPs we continued to volunteer at Hospice after our graduation; I maintained my position as an FNP, and Robin was hired to be the therapeutic musician for the local hospital.

What is this work we do? History is replete with answers, if not explanations. In the

Old Testament Book of Samuel, the young David plays his harp for the tormented Saul: evil spirits were said to depart from the king as the music flowed. Plato writes, "Music gives a soul to the universe, wings to the mind, flight to the imagination, and life to everything."

Modern scientific studies show strong evidence that therapeutic music can result in a range of benefits: reduced blood pressure and anxiety, stabilized heart rates, elevated endorphin levels, and improved cognition and sleep patterns, among others. In his 2007 bestseller, *Musicophilia*, the late renowned neurologist Dr. Oliver Sacks described his patients' reactions to music: the Parkinson's patient who becomes animated when stimulated by music; the agitated Alzheimer's patient who calms after musical exposure; the stroke victim, unable to speak, who finds words while hearing music.

Robin's experiences offering live, bedside therapeutic music in varied settings to the ill, the elderly, and the dying offer a rare view into the responses of patients, staff, family, friends, clinicians. She uses her gifts as an agent of holistic healing, adapting to the unique and changing needs of each patient. (I remember many of the persons she writes about because I also played music for them.) Many people asked us how we could work in these settings, thinking, suggesting that it must be depressing. But Robin show us that death, serious illness, and aging need not be feared as enemies of living, but can be embraced as opportunities for celebration, growth, vision as we tilt toward the natural conclusion of our lives.

I hope you enjoy the chapters in *Musical Morphine* as much as I did, and derive new meaning from what it means to travel in the circle of life.

Susan E. Casler

MS, FNP-BC, ACHPN, CMP

NB: Casler's experiences at Hospice steered her toward palliative care. She earned a post-Master's certificate in Palliative Care thorough Ursuline College and currently, works as a Palliative Care Nurse Practitioner at the Veterans' Administration Medical Center in Albany, N.Y., as a member of a multi disciplinary team. "Every day I have the honor of helping America's soldiers through serious illness: prescribing medication for comfort, listening empathically, or reviewing care options with deep sensitivity."

Introduction

I came to write *Musical Morphine: Transforming Pain One Note at a Time* because it would not let me go. When I told people of my work as a Certified Music Practitioner, trained to offer live, one-on-one bedside music to the critically and chronically ill, the elderly, and the dying, over and over I heard, "You ought to write about this."

It was both easy and difficult to do so. The stories in this book are so alive for me that now, when I re-read them, I still enjoy reacquainting myself with the people, the places, and the events I have described. (Most names have been changed, but others have been used with permission.) As characters in a story, and as individuals I have known and cared about, they remain part of my life.

- How could I ever forget Dolores's desire to live until Christmas? And Helen's cussing up a storm?
- Did deaf, ninety-six-year-old Lillian really hear the harp?
- How did Kurt, dying of acute heart disease, end up singing on stage?
- Ron, the young Marine, declined music, but I sang anyway. Did I do the right thing?

Two-and-a-half years of preparation for certification as a music practitioner, plus a decade as a practicing CMP, have inspired and informed my life as no other activity has. But the work itself, as rewarding as it is, can be difficult to undertake. Why do I feel called to follow this difficult, often unsavory path? And what have I learned?

CMPs offer live, one-on-one bedside music to the critically and chronically ill, the elderly, and the dying; we are considered complementary or integrative healthcare providers. Music for Healing and Transition, Inc., the organization with which I trained and the only one offering board-standards certification, backs all its teaching with current research from physcians and scientists examining the effects of music on humans across a wide spectrum of age, gender, and wellness.

This work is also a form of palliative care, the underutilized, misunderstood medical specialty that seeks to make patients more comfortable, nothing else. Unlike its reputation for only end-of-life care, palliative care makes the rounds to patients who likely will recover from illness or surgery: it attends every age and stage on the life-to-death spectrum. Music is a valuable tool in this corner of medicine.

Becoming a CMP is not a path that's easily discovered or easily followed. Patients and practitioners alike have their individual musical heritage, preferences, and abilities and talents. My music has taken me from the concert hall of the Kennedy Center in Washington, DC, where I sang classical music with the Fairfax Choral Society, to the hand-built outdoor stage at Colvin Run Mill Park in Great Falls, Virginia, singing and playing "old-timey" music with the Mill Run Dulcimer Band. I have sung in church choirs, performed at schools and parties, recorded black vinyl and CDs in the studio, taught all levels of guitar and dulcimer, and made music casually with friends and family. I run deep and wide with my music, a huge asset that I share with patients from all walks of life.

As a teenager, I wanted to be a doctor. There weren't many female physicians in my life, either practicing medicine or entering medical school, in the 1960s when I was exploring my options for college. My parents doubted I could manage difficult math and science requirements to be a physician—they also cited their inability to pay for medical school. So, despite my innate interest in a healing career, I crossed "doctor" off my list of possible professions.

I considered making music my major. Instead I was lucky to be born into a musical family and took for granted my ease with learning and performing instrumental and vocal music both from written scores and by ear. My mother had earned a degree in vocal and piano music and presumed I would follow in her footsteps. That did not occur, in part because of my rebellion against the rigidity of formal music training: the established notion that "a musician" must study and incorporate music theory in order to play, and the insistence on reading music note by note. I was gifted with the ability to improvise easily, as well as to play by ear any music I heard. My mother—and formal music schools—had no place for me and my style of music-making: in their eyes I was not "a real musician." Therefore, I scratched "music major" from my list of options.

I ended up studying English literature as an undergraduate, and psychology and counseling in graduate school, becoming a teacher and then a counselor in secondary education.

By chance, or fate, my early interest in medicine and my gifts in music, along with the skills of careful communication that I learned and practiced as a teacher and counselor, came together seamlessly in my work as a CMP. Together, those attributes contribute mightily to my ability to deliver empathic, compassionate service as a music practitioner to the ill and dying. Even my own personal health issues have taught me that self-advocacy, being heard when you tell your medical narrative, and keeping abreast of health information, are necessary for achieving wellness. Like many of us, I am the sum total of all my parts, lucky to have found a special place in this world.

Musical Morphine, too, is the sum total of many parts. The book began as one story, then another—just a compilation of short vignettes about patient encounters—written mostly as a journal to process what went on after I delivered music. When I first read them to members of my small writing group, the response was overwhelming, gradually leading to my decision to gather the stories into a book.

That decision is due to passion—for patients, for caregivers, for families and friends experiencing illness, decline, and death, and faced with an extraordinarily complex medical system. As I circulate through the halls of hospices, hospitals, nursing homes, rehab centers, clinics, and private homes, I am moved to pass on what I learn in hopes that readers will benefit, just as I have.

Who among us will not be the caregiver, or the cared-for, at some stage in our lives? If *Musical Morphine* allows you to face the inevitable dilemmas of being human with newfound wisdom, love, courage, compassion, then my work and my passion will, I hope, have proved their worth.

Robin Russell Gaiser

January 2016

Table of Contents

Dedication

I dedicate this book to my husband, Gordon Leo Gaiser, who heard the early drafts of every chapter in this book; and to all therapeutic musicians, Certified Music Practitioners, and Music Therapists; and to others whose work brings peace and improved quality of life to the dying and suffering.

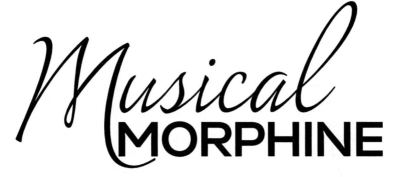

Musical MORPHINE

Transforming Pain
One Note at a Time

Chapter 1

Throw Me in for One Last Dip

My father was dying.

On a whim I brought my guitar to the hospital and sang and played for him.

He was drugged, yet still in severe pain, confused, disoriented. But I noticed something curious happening each time I offered him music.

His hands, wrinkled and blotchy, his taut knuckles clutching the bed railings, loosened their grip. His shoulders and chest, held rigidly in place against his discomfort, relaxed. His wispy breathing deepened and slowed.

I saw his contorted face yield to a soft expression and his eyes close as he descended into a restful, welcome sleep. On occasion, he sang with me, smiling with the recognition of so many tunes he had taught me.

Did he respond because I was his daughter, because I knew his favorite music?

Probably.

But there was something more.

~~

My husband Gordon and I had recently relocated from northern Virginia to rural upstate New York, where we purchased my parents' retirement home in the Adirondack Mountains. It was late June. Their two-and-a-half acres by the Great Sacandaga Lake held a restored 1863 farmhouse, a two-story Dutch barn, and an in-ground pool. Everything was fed by artesian well water from a bubbling spring a quarter-mile up the hill from the house. When we moved in, my parents were already situated in a smaller, brand-new house on the lake in the village of Northville, population one thousand. We were now three miles apart, rather than four hundred and sixty.

My father wept when we agreed to buy the lake house: it was hard for him to sell this treasure to just anyone. My mother heaved a sigh of relief, since its upkeep required constant attention. For the past seven years they had been occupied with keeping my father alive rather than tending the old house and acreage.

My mother amazed me with her constant care of my father. She kept a low profile when it came to death and illness, but with Dad she traded her life of music, bridge, Tai Chi, church work, and friends for unrelenting doctor's appointments, emergency room visits, transportation to dialysis, and supremely unsavory nursing duties keeping him clean, fed, and medicated.

She was not at all a caregiver when it came to me and my brothers; she considered our illnesses an inconvenience. I recall being left home alone around the age of eight with double ear infections while she took off in the car to who knows where. My ear drums ruptured, and when she returned home, her home remedy was to stuff cotton and warm olive oil into my raging ears.

Going to the doctor cost money. Saving money was a theme in my mother's life story. Perhaps that factored in to her solo home care of my father.

"The barn needs painting," Mom said. She didn't need to tell us. We knew how high the grass covering the open fields had become, so that even the path to the beach was overgrown. Spider webs and clusters of ladybugs clung to the corners of the rooms in the house, and a film over the windows that looked out at the lake made a sunny day look cloudy. The flower gardens were weedy and unkempt, and storm windows still hugged the screens of the old front porch.

Gordon and I got to work unpacking and cleaning, mowing, repairing the house and restoring the grounds. A barn full of Dad's tools and machinery greeted Gordon, who began nursing the mower, the snowblower, the edger, the leaf grinder, and the chainsaw back to health. I called my dad one day to invite him and Mom over to the house.

"Dad, are you up to coming over? The raspberries are all ripe and I'll get some ice cream."

"Rob, that would be great," he answered. His failed kidneys and years of dialysis didn't allow ice cream in his diet, but I knew his condition was so deteriorated that a little ice cream made no difference at this point.

Gordon and I picked my parents up at their house, loaded Dad's wheelchair into the trunk, and drove out to the lake house.

"Oh, the yard looks beautiful. You two have really worked hard," Mom said. I had weeded, then planted orange and yellow marigolds surrounding red salvia in her favorite front garden.

Even before Gordon turned off the car engine Dad said rather unexpectedly, "I'd like to go in the barn one more time." Gordon had left the barn doors wide open, creating an enticing, irresistible invitation. He lowered Dad into his wheelchair and pushed him over the bumpy grass into the barn and switched on the light. Mom and I followed.

"Gordon, look what you've done!" The order, the cleanly swept interior caught Dad's attention.

"Sit right there," said Gordon. One by one he pushed or carried each piece of machinery out to the center of the barn floor.

"They look all cleaned up," Dad said. "Do they run?"

Gordon smiled and pulled the starter cord on the big mower. Soon the old engine pounded away, sending gray smoke and gasoline fumes into the air.

Dad shook his head, his eyes sparkled. He smiled his crooked smile out of the corner of his mouth. One by one Gordon started each machine until an entire symphony of repaired engines roared their sweet sounds into the barn and beyond. It was music to Dad's ears. Mom and I watched the interplay of both men delighting in the timbre and smells of old equipment.

After the engine concert we wheeled Dad around to the deck that overlooked the pool, now pristine and clear, and the open lake with three small islands where dad had watched eagles' nests through his binoculars. I delivered heaping bowls of ice cream covered with the raspberries I'd picked from the patch beside the barn earlier in the afternoon. We sat in the waning light spooning in mouthfuls of dessert as sailboats slid by in the evening breeze. Orange, blue, and peach colored the sky as the sun eased behind the mountains across the lake. No one interrupted the silence. This was Dad's favorite spot and likely his last chance to enjoy it.

Not long after that, my father lost the last of his mobility. His legs were riddled with festering open sores as his vascular system failed. Strong narcotic pain medication no longer worked, and his toes and feet blackened with the creep of gangrene.

At one point my cousin, who is a nurse, and I were enlisted by Dad's visiting nurse to learn how to tend his wounds. My mother didn't even enter the bedroom while the nurse taught us how to remove his bandages, clean, medicate, and re-dress his legs: this was way out of her comfort zone. I coaxed myself through the awful process as he writhed in pain, trying to preserve his dignity and express his gratitude for my efforts. I could not stand to see my father in such misery at my hand. After two days of this routine, I knew this was out of my comfort zone, too.

None of his doctors had examined him in three weeks, and he needed to be seen. My mother stood in the background as I made the call to his renal specialist's office. I was directed to get him to the local emergency room where the doctor would meet us. Mom receded into the background even more as I called 911 to transport him to the hospital. I sat on Dad's bedside, holding his hand as we waited for the ambulance. I had never seen his eyes so full of fear.

"Do I have to go by ambulance? Can't we just go in the car?"

"I'm afraid getting you in and out of the car would be too painful for you. And it's hard for us to move you." I think he knew this might be his last ride. He wanted to go quietly in the family car. "I asked the dispatcher to please silence the siren."

"Thanks." He turned his head to the wall. I think he might have been crying.

Once the doctor unbandaged Dad's legs in the emergency room, he hastily arranged for Dad to be rushed to Albany Medical Center, nearly two hours away from Northville, for emergency surgery. It was hours before the transportation arrived, and during that time his pain medicines were neglected, despite my reports to medical attendants that he was in severe distress. Eventually he was given morphine, but the small dose did nothing to calm him.

By this time he was frantic, pulling at the bedrails trying to get out and walk, trying to escape the pain like a caged animal caught in a trap. I was scared and furious. My rage overflowed onto the nurse with a heated request for more pain medication. An oral medication was given and he settled some. Finally, he was loaded into another ambulance for delivery to Albany Med. Gordon, Mom, and I hurried behind the medical transport. When we finally arrived it was past eleven p.m.

~~

As I sat in the surgery waiting room, thoughts of my father came and went, along with my cousin's recent remark. "We call him the unofficial mayor of Northville. Everyone knows him and loves him." I recalled trips to the village Post Office with him. He greeted everyone by name, hugged them, kissed the women and kids, shook hands with the men, patted their shoulders, remembered their stories. What would have been a fifteen-minute event extended to over an hour, a ritual I came to enjoy. Northville was his ancestral home, a place where he contributed, where he mattered.

Dad was tall, trim, a spiffy dresser. He had black curly hair and dark eyes, truly a handsome man. Women his age still clucked about what a hunk he was in his day.

"I was in love with him. I sat by my window every day to watch him walk by in his uniform on his way to his job at the Adirondack Inn," said Connie, a church friend and lifelong resident of the village. She and my Aunt Nan were still best friends. Dad was only four years older than Connie when he became bell captain at the inn. He met my mother there during the summer of 1940. She was the gorgeous new waitress and singer in the dining room: they were both sixteen. As children on vacation in Northville, we were always driven to the exact spot under a large oak tree near the inn where Dad kissed Mom for the first time. From the back seat we watched Dad take Mom in his arms, then they'd giggle and smooch for what seemed like a long time.

I remembered his love of water skiing. He invariably wore a white terry-cloth hat and held his pipe in his mouth while zipping back and forth across the wake, dropping one ski to slalom, smiling all the while. After undergoing bypass surgery, he made sure he was back on the skis the next summer.

~~

"We'll try to save his leg," said the surgeon before the operation. "But it's very far gone."

Two hours later the same man walked over to where we waited. We stood up. "I'm sorry, but we had to amputate just below the knee," he said. I closed my eyes, caught my breath, felt tears dripping down my cheeks. Dad would never waterski or walk again. With that statement his stature, his dignity, his image vanished.

To me, this was the day my father died.

All three of my brothers and their wives traveled to Albany Medical Center to be with Dad after his surgery. The six of them, along with Gordon, Mom, and me, circled around his hospital bed. We had planned to say good-bye, to give Dad permission to let go. Glenn, my oldest brother, was the chosen spokesman.

We held hands as he spoke. Most of us had tears in our eyes. "Dad, we're all here to support you and we love you. Thank you for being a solid provider for us. But we want you to know that you have suffered enough and if …"

Dad, fidgeting in his bed, his eyes darting around the room, avoiding eye contact with any of us, interrupted. "Anyone got any Necco Wafers?"

Glenn remained silent. We shifted our weight, looked around at each other, until finally the uncomfortable silence gave way to laughing and wiping tears. Dad was not at all ready to hear about dying. I had, of course, stashed his beloved Necco Wafers in his bedside table. He put out his hand, and I dropped one green and one brown one, his favorites, into his waiting palm. He smiled.

"Mmmmmm. Thanks." And that was that.

During his stay at Albany Medical Center, a large teaching hospital, hordes of doctors and residents rotated in and out of his room, poked and prodded him, asked and re-asked him questions. Even a prosthetics specialist sat us down to discuss making a new leg for him. All these strangers added to his growing disorientation. Often he asked where he was, when he could go home, if he could take a walk. Mom, Gordon, and I glanced back and forth at each other and wondered just whom this exuberant salesman was talking about; he had been too weak to walk even before his leg was removed. This was crazy.

Late at night two days after surgery, Dad's blood pressure plunged so low that a Code Blue was called. Medical personnel swarmed to his room and revived him. The hospital called my mother the next morning to report the incident: she still had his medical power of attorney. With no Do Not Resuscitate (DNR) order in place, I began to realize how little my parents had talked or planned about their deaths, their end-of-life care. My mother reported to me that as Dad was being loaded on the stretcher to go to Albany, he told her, through his pain and drowsiness, "I guess I'll have to give up the lead." She had no idea what he meant. I wondered if he was saying he was ready to die.

With all this uncertainty I knew I needed to get Mom to the Elder Care attorney I had heard about thorough my friend Barbara. When Barb's own father became terminally ill, her mother—like mine—was under-prepared financially, medically, and legally. This attorney's expertise, along with his kindness and compassion, had saved the day, and had even become a source of emotional support for her and her mother. I liked the sound of that.

The final straw with the big teaching medical center came for me when a young gastroenterologist reported that Dad had some rectal bleeding. "I've ordered a colonoscopy," he said matter-of-factly. I stepped back, put my hand up to stop him.

"My mother and I need to talk. Hold the procedure until I get back to you."

I took Mom into the waiting area. "Don't you think this is crazy?" I asked her.

She looked perplexed; she had always followed a doctor's advice. But hesitantly she said, "Well, I guess so. I hate to see your father go through anything more."

"And for what? Mom, he's dying."

I was stunned by my own words. She began to weep. I was too busy making plans in my mind for the next step in my father's care to let my emotions take over. I reached over and took my mother's hand, then said, "Let's get him back to St. Mary's in Amsterdam where he knows the staff. Enough of this."

We transferred Dad from Albany to a local hospital, where he could take dialysis and be closer to us for daily visits—and where my ritual of playing and singing music for him began. Sometimes patients with walkers or in wheelchairs congregated outside his room and stayed as long as there was music. Other patients and visitors poked their heads into his room as my music escaped into the halls of the hospital.

"Can you stop in next door?" a visitor said. "My mother could really use some music."

"I wish all our patients could hear this," the nurses often said.

I began to wonder if something more was going on, to realize that I was not just a daughter singing her father's favorite songs.

Dad's health declined to the point where dialysis was no longer effective. I knew of a Mountain Valley Hospice in the next larger town and called to inquire about their services. I knew very little about what they did other than having heard they dealt well with end-of-life patients. Their explanations and responses to my questions, their compassion and understanding, assured me that they would be an asset to my family as we moved through Dad's dying process.

At this point Mom, exhausted and shocked that her husband of fifty-seven years was actually dying, had readily turned the details over to me—

now that we lived in Northville. For it was another theme in her life to rely on me for difficult decisions. As the oldest of four, and the only girl, my role as "the responsible one" had been established early on, so I easily, almost automatically, slid into this position as lead caregiver for my father.

Gordon and I discussed options and finally agreed to offer our house, the beloved lake house, as a location for Dad to receive Hospice care. His favorite spot had been the knotty-pine-paneled room with windows on three sides offering views of the lake and pool, the grounds and gardens. I had decorated it with rustic-style furniture and accessories when we moved in. Gordon and I called it the Adirondack Room.

Mom liked our offer. She and I chose a day when Dad was lucid to propose the change to Hospice to him. It meant giving up dialysis and facing a short window of time until his body succumbed and he died. I waffled about how to offer this suggestion. I never wanted him to think I was trying to hasten his death.

"Dad, it looks like dialysis isn't making you feel better anymore." His large brown eyes met mine then looked back at my mother who was seated behind me. I reached under the bed railing and took his hand.

"Gordon and I want to offer you the opportunity to come home to the lake house to the Adirondack Room, with Hospice." I swallowed hard, then proceeded, "You know," I said resisting the urge to look away, "this means giving up dialysis."

Dad sat very still, and stared into my eyes. He remained silent.

"Just think about it. You don't have to give an answer today." He nodded. "You have other options, too," I said. "You could continue the dialysis and stay here in the hospital. Or you could move to a Hospice room in this hospital and quit dialysis. But be assured Gordon and I are honestly offering the lake house."

Then he spoke. "How would you manage?" He was speaking directly to me, making sure I could handle the stress, the care, the emotional drain. He knew me well. Ever my protector.

"Dad, thanks for asking. We discussed that and we'd hire round-the-clock private nursing assistance."

He looked away. I squeezed his hand. "Think about it."

The next morning I was awakened by the phone at 8 a.m. It was my mother. "Robin, the hospital just called, and your father's refusing dialysis and says he's leaving the hospital today."

"Oh, no. We're not ready. Can you tell him to hold off, take dialysis? We'll get the house ready as soon as we can." Without dialysis, he could die before he got his wish to go home.

"I'll try," she said, and hung up.

Gordon and I went into action. I called Hospice to start the admitting procedure while he removed pieces of furniture from the Adirondack Room to make space for the hospital bed, the oxygen concentrator, and the supplies Dad would need to come home: bed linens and pads, adult diapers, lotion, drinking straws, moistened wipes. Fall was Dad's favorite season, so I decorated the room with yellow and maroon mums and small pumpkins.

That afternoon Gordon, Mom, and I sat together in Dad's hospital room as the Hospice social worker and nurse completed the intake papers. Two days later Dad arrived by ambulance at the lake house. I still regret how long that took and that he had to endure more dialysis, but in that time relatives made travel plans and arrived to receive him when the ambulance maneuvered by the big birch tree and into our side yard.

I will never forget how alert he was, and how happy. As the EMTs rolled his stretcher by the swimming pool and up onto the deck, he raised his head up off the pillow to take a look and joked, "You might as well throw me in the pool for one last dip." We were astounded at his awareness, his intact humor. With that remark, he eased our grief as we ushered him into the last paragraph of his life.

I would like to say that things went smoothly, as planned. But right away I learned that home care nurses were hard to come by: there was unstaffed time in Dad's round-the-clock care. My brother Glenn and his son, Derek, a chiropractor, drove up from Norfolk, VA to help out. Derek's ease with tending his grandfather was a huge help, but there were still care gaps I could not mange by myself. Mom was hosting Glenn and Derek at her house, and they often lingered over coffee and bagels in the morning before they drove over to the lake house. One such morning a paid caregiver did not show up, nor did anyone else: mother, brother, or nephew. Dad's pain level was increasing, as were his symptoms of congestive heart failure. He had been taking pills easily, but this morning he could not swallow well enough to get one down. I dispatched my husband to the village to buy applesauce to ease the pills down, as instructed by the Hospice nurse; while Gordon was making the grocery run (a six-mile round trip), Dad began to choke and cough. He was having difficulty breathing, so, in a panic, I called my neighbor, who had been a nurse, praying she would pick up the phone.

I blurted out, "I think my Dad's choking to death. I'm alone. Can you come down?"

I watched her rush down the hillside to our side door, where she let herself in and, huffing and puffing, came to the Adirondack room. She raised the back of the hospital bed so Dad was more upright and massaged his back and then his chest. His distress eased ever so slightly. Gordon returned with the applesauce, and she instructed me to crush the pills and add them to a tablespoon of the soft, sweet fruit. I handed her the spoon and observed her well-trained, professional approach: as she talked calmly to Dad, telling him what she was doing, she slipped incremental offerings of the concoction between his lips. He was able to swallow the small portions.

"Didn't Hospice leave you with a liquid medication kit?" she asked, while still working with Dad. "I think the next time he is due for meds he ought to have them from the kit."

I felt stupid. The "kit" was in the refrigerator, placed there by the Hospice nurse after she explained its use, but in my panic I'd forgotten about it. Besides that, I was not at all comfortable measuring and administrating liquid morphine to my father on my own. Where was that home care nurse? And where was my family? Finally I simply wept. Maybe I wasn't equipped to do this.

I had brought Dad home to spend his last days surrounded by his family, our love, and, yes, music. But during all this time, the only music I was able to play for him was Mozart on the stereo.

~~

Our daughter drove over from college for the weekend to see her dear grandfather. They had always shared a bond of special affection, and I cried along with them when she said good-bye. Other family, friends, and neighbors filed by his bed over the five days he remained alive. On a dark, drizzly Sunday our preacher and family gathered around him for a Communion service. He sipped sanctified grape juice with a straw and slowly ate the little white bread cube. I played and sang.

Amazing grace, how sweet the sound, that saved a wretch like me. Everyone joined in, then spontaneously held hands. I think I saw Dad's lips moving with the lyrics.

I once was lost, but now I'm found, was blind but now I see. He fell asleep in the music.

He died two days later in the wee hours of the night, facing the lake, after all of us had gone to bed for some badly needed rest. His favorite Hospice caregiver knocked softly on Gordon's and my bedroom door.

"He's gone," she said. I leapt out of bed.

"I wanted to be with him."

She put her arm around me as we walked to the Adirondack Room. "He chose to go this way."

It took me a nearly a year to understand this concept, to accept it.

Then I got it.

Of course. Dad, my protector to the very end.

Chapter 2

Is This Music Program a Hoax?

I was lost.

Dad was gone and I felt empty. Gordon and I assimilated easily into our new community, joined my parents' church, kept busy with the old house, the huge yard and the machinery. I sang in the tiny church choir directed by my mother, enjoyed extended family gatherings, and visited with my ninety-seven-year-old grandmother, who lived nearby in the family homestead.

I bought a kayak, swam in our pool, walked on our country road, volunteered for the fledgling arts organization, and played old-time music with an elderly Adirondack woman. Still something was missing. The itch to find a new calling remained unsettled. Leaving my career and the hustle-bustle of the metropolitan Washington, DC area was finally settling in.

In the fall I accepted substitute teaching jobs at Northville Central School, but after many years of working as an English teacher, music teacher, and high school guidance counselor, I decided I'd done my stint in education. Subbing was not for me.

A new church friend told me about a yoga class starting, then invited me to go. I went. Standing outside the Veterans of Foreign Wars building after yoga she offered me a stack of old *Yoga Journals.*

"I'm done with these," she said. "You might enjoy some of the articles."

"Thanks," I said taking the magazines from her more out of politeness than interest.

That evening I began flipping through the journals, not really reading anything in particular. I did notice the photos of ultra-slim women wearing gorgeous yoga outfits, twisted into pretzel poses. This magazine isn't for me, I thought.

Then I stopped at an ad. It outlined a certification program for becoming a music practitioner. I read and reread the copy. "Music for Healing and Transition Program." Was this some light-weight training, some fly-by-night bunch eager to take my money for a no-matter certificate? And what was a music practitioner anyway? Since this was an outdated issue of the magazine, was the organization already out of business? Where were classes held? How much did it cost?

With my head buzzing I raced up the stairs to my computer and typed in the web address. Up popped a sophisticated website that answered nearly all my questions. It sounded too good to be true, but this venue seemed to be exactly what I was looking for. With both skepticism and excitement I sent for materials. Until the bulky brown envelope arrived in my mailbox, I spent many a wakeful night rehashing what I'd read on the Internet. And I prayed. *Okay, God, if this is what I'm meant to do, then make it happen.*

Doubt disappeared when I opened the envelope and read the student handbook cover to cover. Graduates were called Certified Music Practitioners.

"Hon, I think I've found a program I want to enroll in," I said to my husband. "Listen to this. A Certified Music Practitioner provides live bedside music to the critically and chronically ill, the elderly and dying."

He looked up from his book. "What would you do with that?" he asked.

"I don't know yet." Both my bachelors and masters degrees were taken with solid career goals in mind. Saying I had no plan in place felt liberating.

I thought back to my father: his beautifully relaxed face, his open hands resting by his sides, his unlabored breathing, his singing with me when I offered him music over the last months of his life. The mission and message of Music for Healing and Transition, Inc. legitimized my gut feelings that there was more to my music-making than entertainment or distraction.

The only flaw in the application I received was the limited space available for detailing my musical experience. I would have to add an extra page to include all the musical instruments I played, the bands I was in, the many CDs I'd recorded, my membership in the classical choral society. I wanted the folks who reviewed my application to know I composed, arranged, taught, performed. And maybe most important, that I memorized music easily, played by ear as well as read music, and improvised effortlessly. I hoped my passion for music would come through.

At last I folded the application and two letters of recommendation into a return envelope and rushed to the Post Office. As I stuffed the envelope into the mail slot I worried whether my not having a degree in music might hurt my chances of admission.

Two weeks later, an acceptance letter arrived—along with an award for a partial scholarship granted for musical knowledge and experience. This felt right!

Classes were taught all over the United States, including some a mere two hours away in Hillsdale, New York. I couldn't wait to share my good news, especially with a new music friend who was a nurse practitioner.

"Sue, I just got accepted into a Certified Music Practitioner program called Music for Healing and Transition. I'm going to start classes. Have you ever heard of it?"

Her reply stunned me. "You're not going to believe this. I've been thinking about applying myself. I heard about MHTP two years ago from a harpist in Saratoga," she said. "She's a CMP."

"You're kidding. Let's do this together. How about you apply?"

"I'll think about it," she said, "but with a full-time job it could be tricky."

But without any more nudging from me, Sue applied and was also accepted. I was overjoyed, not least at the prospect of sharing the driving, especially in winter months, the costs of required books, and overnights in motels for weekend class modules. This was really feeling right.

Over the next eighteen months Sue and I traveled back and forth to Hillsdale for eighty hours of classes, read ten books each, and enjoyed spirited discussions about the information accumulating in our heads and binders. I was especially impressed that so much scientific research backed up the teaching about how music affected patients. The quizzes, book reports, repertoire notebooks, seventeen-page final exam, and clinical practicum at a regional medical center thoroughly prepared us for the forty-five-hour internship which lay ahead. After interning, we would each need to submit a thirty-minute recording to our advisors using our accumulated repertoire to demonstrate our knowledge of what music to employ for various patient conditions. Once a final summary report was written, we would receive our badges—with "Certified Music Practitioner" imprinted below our names.

As friends and family learned of my pursuit, many cringed at the thought of being in the midst of the dying, the sick, the desperate, the demented. My mother shook her head. Yet I felt called to be there. I knew I could offer myself and my music.

I recalled my earlier prayer. *If this is what I'm meant to do, then make it happen.*

It was happening.

Chapter 3

Welcome to Hospice House

"They've never had music and they've never heard of a Certified Music Practitioner," Sue told me over the phone. "But they accepted us." With my required shots, TB test, Hospice training, and paperwork completed, my internship was really going to happen.

I don't remember driving the twenty-five miles from the lake house to Mountain Valley Hospice for my first day of my internship. With nervous anticipation, I pulled into the freshly lined parking lot facing the front entry. The brand-new eight-bed, in-patient house had just opened its doors in Gloversville, New York. From the outside the building and grounds were stunning: I could have mistaken it for a ski lodge. As I walked up to the entrance, I noticed stained glass windows in both side panels surrounding the heavy oak door. A small engraved plaque near the door handle read, "In honor of Nancy Dowd, founder of Mountain Valley Hospice House." Nudging the weighty door open with a guitar and a loaded satchel in my hand alerted the receptionist, who came around her desk to help me.

"Can I carry anything? You must be the new intern," she said.

"Thanks, I think I can handle it if you hold the door. This place is gorgeous."

"We're very proud of it."

"Hi." I smiled. "I'm Robin, and I'm one of the MHTP interns." I had already fastened my badge to my blouse and looped the lanyard with my Hospice ID around my neck. They were hiding under my coat. But I still felt official. And welcomed.

"Let me take you around a little bit and then we'll go to the patient wing so you can meet Kathleen, our head nurse." We walked slowly, passing a library with well-stocked, built-in floor-to-ceiling wood bookcases, flanked by comfy-looking blue wing chairs and wooden end tables topped with leaded stained glass lamps. "Make sure you help yourself to any of the books and the Hospice literature," she said.

A conference room held a long glossy table with yellow suede chairs placed around the perimeter. Down the hall was a great room with wooden beams angled to support a high cathedral ceiling dotted with skylights. A natural stone fireplace soared to the top of the ceiling and a long hearth beckoned someone to sit by the fire. Stained wood dominated the open space, which looked out to a patio through a wall of French doors to dense woods. The furnishings were inviting, plush, and cozy. I wondered if I'd ever sit down in this room.

We turned left to enter the patient wing. I was struck by how quiet it was, how the warm sage-green carpeting and wall colors gave off an aura of calm, a sense of refreshment. I could feel some of my nervousness vanishing in this setting. A dark-haired, middle-aged woman in a nurse's outfit sat at the spacious nurses' station midway down the wide hallway. When she saw us she stood up, smiled, and held out her hand.

"Welcome to the House. We're so eager for you to join the team. I think music will be so special here. I'm Kathleen, one of the nurses." We shook hands and I felt an immediate rapport with her.

I introduced myself, adding, "I must admit I'm a little nervous today.

But I can't wait to get started." I glanced up and down the patient hall. "Are you full?"

"Yes, we haven't had an empty bed since we opened."

"How do you want to go about this?" I asked.

She explained that Chris, my supervisor and the volunteer coordinator I would report to, was not there that day.

"Do you think I can still do music today without him?" I asked.

"Yes, absolutely. He has so many other duties, you won't see him much."

"Can you direct me to some patients you think might be candidates for music?"

"Bob," she said without hesitation. "He's isolating himself, walling us all out. He's sitting in the great room."

"Sounds good," I said. "Is there a place for me to unpack my instruments and hang my coat?"

Kathleen pointed to an open floor space next to a window behind the nurses' station.

"Thanks, I'll get started." She returned to her desk and her paperwork, while I moved over to the open space and removed my guitar from its case, hung my coat on a wobbly rack, adjusted my name badges, and walked down the wide hall.

I stopped at the door leading into the great room, squared my shoulders, took a deep breath, and stood there. MHTP classes taught me to park my ego at the door and enter only after reviewing a series of steps calling forth my desire to be of service, the need to become centered, to have no expectations, and to maintain an open mind. I took more breaths as I rehearsed these ideas. Then I asked for guidance from God. I visualized the door frame as a halo of love that blessed me as I stepped into the unknown space. Going into the room of a dying patient, a complete stranger, oddly reminded me of making cold calls when I was a newspaper ad salesperson. Suddenly I felt awkward, uncomfortable. How would I be received?

I opened the door and walked in. A man was seated alone on a long floral-print sofa facing the blazing fireplace. His crisp blue button-down shirt under a maroon cardigan sweater, his brown corduroy slacks, and his horn-rimmed glasses led me to think he was an employee. Then I noticed how pale and thin he was, how his eyes looked tired and lifeless.

I spoke. "Hi, Bob. I'm Robin, the new therapeutic music intern here at the house." He didn't say a word. "I'm wondering if you'd like some soothing music this afternoon. This is not a concert. And if you've had enough, I'll stop any time. The music is designed to help you rest, relax, feel better."

I could see him eyeing the guitar and scrutinizing me from head to toe. He had a bit of a scowl on his face. I imagined him thinking, "Oh boy, here we go with 'Kum Ba Yah'." I waited for a flat "no-thank-you."

Instead, he said, "I like classical music," rather emphatically.

"I can do that," I said. "Will you give me a try? And if it isn't what you want, I'll gladly leave, no questions asked, no hurt feelings."

"Okay," he said, but I felt his hesitation, saw him look down and cross his arms over his chest.

I sat near him and began a classical style accompaniment on my guitar and then added my low-pitched alto voice humming the Largo movement from Dvorak's *New World Symphony*. When the last note ended he motioned for me to continue, so I moved on to Sibelius's *Finlandia*, then the "Ode to Joy" from Beethoven's *Ninth Symphony*. He unfolded his arms and put his head back to rest on the sofa, and a pleasant expression came over his face. I closed out our session with "Jesu, Joy of Man's Desiring," continuing to merely hum the melodies with my guitar playing. When I finished he smiled and sighed.

"Have you had enough?" I said.

"Maybe for today, but you can come back," he said, raising his head and looking at me.

"I'm glad you liked it."

"I did," he said.

Bob became an avid fan of all kinds of my music over the next weeks. The nurses told me he asked when I would be coming in and made sure he was dressed and ready for my arrival.

One Saturday I arrived to find him surrounded by his family in the great room. The hospice social worker had briefed me that his adult children weren't speaking to each other and that his wife, often abrupt and grumpy, was disabled and in a wheelchair. Tension permeated the room. No one was talking except Bob and his wife. He looked up when I entered.

"Oh, Robin," he said. Then he turned to the rest of the group. "This is the house musician." No one moved a muscle except to briefly look at me, and then return to their downcast, blank stares. I could feel anxiety creep over me. I wanted to excuse myself; the silence was suffocating.

For some reason I had packed another instrument that day, a rhythm instrument called a limberjack. Wondering how this fit in with MHTP protocol, I hesitated a minute. A limberjack in a hospice setting?

Oh, well, I thought, and slid the little hand-carved wooden man and his thin paddleboard out of my satchel. I sat on the edge of the square wood coffee table, situated the paddle board under my thigh, and began tapping my fingers on the board. I held the limberjack with a long dowel rod fastened to his back over the board so his feet barely touched. His arms and legs, loose and hinged, began to fly around, his feet clicked away in a steady rhythm. I added my voice.

Jim Jim along, Jim along Josie. Jim Jim along, Jim along Joe. I kept my eyes on Bob. This was for him. He was watching me and the limberjack intently. I noticed him motion to one of his sons who got up and disappeared into the adjoining kitchen. I continued. *Dance Jim along, Jim along Josie, Dance Jim along Jim along Joe.*

The son returned and handed his father two silver tablespoons. Bob, who was now wheelchair-bound like his wife, arranged the spoons between his fingers and began a clickety-clack in perfect rhythm to the limberjack's tapping and my singing.

Everyone's eyes turned to Bob. One of the daughters pulled a camera from her purse and began snapping pictures. The sons sat forward on their chairs; their facial expressions softened and their shoulders relaxed. I felt the heavy atmosphere begin to dissipate. I made up several extra verses to the funny folk song to prolong this precious time for Bob's family. *Hop Jim along; Jump Jim along; Laugh Jim along,* and so it went.

When the music stopped Bob spoke. "Boys, get me out of this wheelchair and over to the coffee table. I want to play that limberjack." What would Hospice and MHTP say to this? I wondered.

Without hesitation the adult sons lifted their dad onto the table's edge and sat on either side of him to ensure his safety. I handed over the limberjack, grabbed my guitar, and off we went.

Buffalo gals won't ya come out tonight, come out tonight, come out tonight, Buffalo gals won't ya come out tonight and dance to the light of the moon. The other daughter got up, took the spoons and joined in. Even Bob's wife smiled at the sight of the family band and its impromptu merrymaking.

When we stopped singing and playing, small conversations started up among family members. I thought this was a good time to excuse myself and allow the family to enjoy their privacy. The atmosphere had changed dramatically.

"You can put the limberjack on the counter of the nurses' station when you're done," I said. "I need to see some other patients this afternoon."

"Thanks," someone said as I excused myself from the room.

I was perplexed. How would I report this experience in my patient notes? I decided I would write about everything. I would tell all. This was definitely healing music at its best, limberjack, spoons, and all.

Bob became bedridden. One morning as I sang and played for him in his room, he blurted out, "When you give me music, I don't feel my pain." Our eyes met. I could hardly continue singing, but I caught my breath and tried not to interrupt the music. Another morning he shared stories about his military service during World War II; how he was on a destroyer in the Pacific. I realized our relationship had deepened. He trusted me. And I also realized playing and singing for him was something more than just music. It was ministry.

Eventually he lapsed into non-responsiveness, a term used in place of unconsciousness. His eyes were shut, but his breathing, although somewhat labored, was regular and steady. Knowing his hearing was intact, I entered his room one late November afternoon, sat beside his bed and sang to him. Just my voice, no instruments. *Eternal father, strong to save, whose arm has bound the restless wave.* I reached for his hand and continued. *Who bade the mighty ocean deep, its own appointed limits keep. Oh hear us when we cry to thee, for those in peril on the sea.* The "Navy Hymn" was one of his favorites.

I felt a weak squeeze to my hand and saw tears form in the corners of his eyes. I knew he was close to his time and I didn't know how much longer I could maintain my composure in his presence. So I sang only that one hymn.

"Bob, I'm going to miss you." I felt another weak squeeze to my hand. I stood up over him, slid my hand out from his. "God bless you, Bob. Have a good journey up." Then I eased my way out of the room.

The next day he died peacefully.

I mourned this first loss of a patient I had served; I dreaded returning to the Hospice House the next week and walking past Bob's empty room. Could I hold myself together to offer healing music to other patients?

When I looked into his room, another patient had already moved in. I stood outside the door remembering the funny limberjack dancing its way into Bob's and his family's hearts, and Bob's initial hesitancy about having music at all. A nurse passed by and patted me gently on the shoulder. With her gesture, I came back to thinking about the day's work ahead of me and slowly walked to my space behind the nurses' station.

I hung up my coat, unpacked my instruments, and moved on.

This wasn't going to be easy work.

Eternal Father, Strong to Save
(The Navy Hymn)

MELITA

William Whiting, 1860, 1869

John B. Dykes, 1861

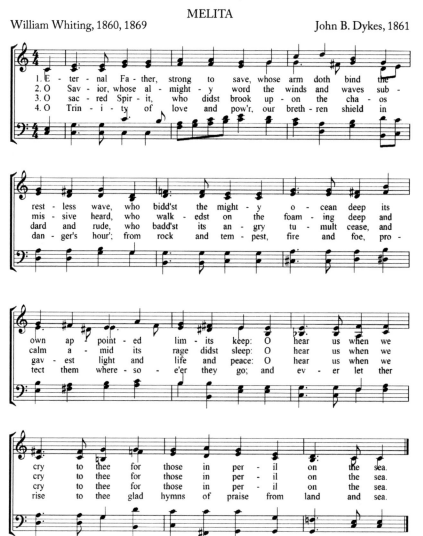

1. E - ter - nal Fa - ther, strong to save, whose arm doth bind the
2. O Sav - ior, whose al - might - y word the winds and waves sub -
3. O sac - red Spir - it, who didst brook up - on the cha - os
4. O Trin - i - ty of love and pow'r, our breth - ren shield in

rest - less wave, who bidd'st the might - y o - cean deep its
mis - sive heard, who walk - edst on the foam - ing deep and
dard and rude, who badd'st its an - gry tu - mult cease, and
dan - ger's hour'; from rock and tem - pest, fire and foe, pro -

own ap - point - ed lim - its keep: O hear us when we
calm a - mid its rage didst sleep: O hear us when we
gav - est light and life and peace: O hear us when we
tect them where - so - e'er they go; and ev - er let ther

cry to thee for those in per - il on the sea.
cry to thee for those in per - il on the sea.
cry to thee for those in per - il on the sea.
rise to thee glad hymns of praise from land and sea.

Chapter 4

Almost Heaven: Lavender and Camo

"Can you and Sue do music for the Christmas party at the House?" Chris asked. He explained that patients and their families, Hospice staff, donors, and Board of Directors with their spouses were all invited. Maybe he thought MHTP interns also provided free entertainment. I let that thought pass since he and Hospice were doing Sue and me a favor.

"Sure," I said. "I'll ask Sue." She readily agreed, and we met twice weekly to prepare a long list of sacred and secular holiday music for the party.

In early December, a new patient was admitted. Dolores, a perky, round, elderly woman occupied a corner room on the hall.

"I've got the best room in the house," she joked when I met her. Indeed it was a premiere room with all the light coming through the extra windows and a bathroom with its own tub and shower. At first she was able to reach that fancy bathroom and use the facilities, though as time passed, she gradually became bedridden.

"Would you like some music?" I asked.

"Christmas is my favorite season," she said. "I love all the holiday music. 'Silent Night' is my favorite song." Turning her head to look out the window, she said with less enthusiasm in her voice, "I hope I make it to December twenty-fifth." Her clarity about her musical preferences and her desire to enjoy every minute of the season made it easy for me to choose what music I would offer her.

Dolores and I blew through holiday repertoire session after session. She knew all the music and words and never wanted me to leave. As we sang she often worked on craft projects, her Christmas gifts to family and friends. Her bedside table drawers were stuffed with felt, fabric, glitter, glue, scissors, and yarn. Her room was decorated to the hilt, without a spare inch for another Christmas garland or woven wall hanging. In one corner, her little lighted Christmas tree sat on a round table skirted with fabric imprinted with snowmen, mittens, and cottages spewing smoke out of their stubby chimneys.

It struck me that Dolores, this delightful north-country woman, would never experience her favorite season again.

"My son brought me that tree," she said, smiling broadly and pointing to the Christmas tree. "He's so good to me."

I knew I had to show her the limberjack. She would get a kick out of seeing him dance to "Jingle Bells." I dressed him up like Santa with a red felt hat and white cotton beard scotch-taped to his wooden head. During his dancing debut his hat and beard fell off and crumpled to the floor. Dolores saw opportunity and dug into her craft drawer to find new felt and a bag of cotton.

"He needs a new wardrobe," she said reaching for her scissors.

Jingle bells, jingle bells, jingle all the way. Oh, what fun it is to ride in a one-horse open sleigh. I sang and danced the limberjack while she expertly cut out a new red hat and sewed a tiny white tufted ball on the top. Then she pulled out a wad of cotton and smoothed it into a long soft beard. When I finished the chorus, I handed her the limberjack and she attached the new hat and beard with double-sided tape.

"He'll dance a lot better now," I said. She winked.

She was proud of her work. I think this generous woman wanted to give back to me, although I never expected it. I danced the limberjack in his new costume over and over for her, and she invariably squinted her eyes and laughed out loud at his funny antics.

The afternoon of the party, a few days before Christmas, Sue and I set up our instruments and music stands for the dinnertime gala. Despite a significant snowfall the great room was packed. The stone fireplace roared, and a festive table ytof catered food filled the back of the room. Families huddled close together singing the familiar holiday music while Sue and I played. Everyone loved the limberjack dancing in his Santa costume. I handed out clusters of little bells strung on red ribbons for folks to shake and jingle to the upbeat music. *Rudolph the red-nosed reindeer had a very shiny nose.* Everyone one knew this one.

Dolores wasn't present. She was dying.

During a break in the musical entertainment I slipped away to the back hallway to check on her. Her little Christmas tree cast a warm glow in the darkened room. The oxygen concentrator clicking on and off with her irregular breathing was the only sound in the deathly silence. She lay under a plush fleece Christmas throw I had never seen in her room before: I guessed her son had placed it over her. I took her hand and bent down over her bed close enough to smell the lavender lotion used to soothe her drying skin, and began singing. *Silent night, holy night, all is calm, all is bright.* I left a long pause before I sang the next line. No one was present but the two of us. I know she heard me sing her favorite carol. It was truly a calm, holy night.

Dolores got her wish and died on Christmas Day. I still dress my limberjack in the costume she crafted for him. Her memory lives on in a small red hat and a fluffy cotton beard.

~~

During the week of the holiday party, but still before Christmas day, I encountered quite another Christmas story. Down the Hospice hall a large, loud family from the mountains crammed themselves into a middle-aged, dying woman's room.

"I've tried to quiet them down and close the door," the social worker said, "but there are so many of them, they just open the door when it gets too hot." This gang didn't take her suggestions well and continued their ruckus. The nurses were beside themselves trying to maintain the usual hushed atmosphere for other patients. I took my chances and stuck my head in the door.

"Would you like some quiet Christmas music?" I was hoping to hush the fracas a bit. A bearded teen made a wisecrack and started laughing uproariously.

"That an electric guitar? We only like loud country," he said looking around for a rise out of the crowd.

"Yeah, got any Dolly Parton?" another male voice chimed in. After his comment I heard chuckles around the room. I looked over to the speaker. He was an overweight, middle-aged man with a camouflage ball cap on his head. He had long scraggly hair. He may have been my patient's husband.

The poor sick woman tried to shush them up, then looked at me with pleading eyes as if she wanted me to discipline them. I could tell she was gravely ill even in the dim light. She was pallid, emaciated. Her nightgown, now too big for her, fell off one shoulder exposing a skeletal upper arm draped in loose flesh. She had very little hair and no eyebrows. Probably from chemo treatments.

Finally, I just stepped into the room, set up my portable chair next to my patient, sat down and began strumming my guitar. "Do you have any favorite Christmas carols?"

No one answered. A woman with long dark hair and big glasses who was dressed in a blue fleece top and a printed holiday turtleneck spoke up. "Can you name some?"

"Joy to the World."

No one responded.

"Oh, Come All Ye Faithful." Silence again.

Then a familiar voice shot out from the back of the room. "How 'bout 'Grandma Got Run Over by a Reindeer'?" It was the same bearded teen. He was probably the dying woman's son. I could see him more clearly now. His camouflage jacket was open over a faded orange T-shirt, and he wore a bright day-glow-orange ball cap. I ignored his comment.

"Do you know 'Silent Night'?" I asked. Surely they would I thought.

The patient nodded her head and a young female voice from the back of the room said she knew the song. I sang one verse accompanied by my guitar and stopped after that. I could tell they were uncomfortable. The men looked back and forth to each other with embarrassed grins; the women sang tentatively. The room was emotionally charged whether they knew it or not. My experience as a counselor told me the joking around, the smart remarks diverted their thoughts away from their underlying fears and the certainty that this woman was near her death.

"Aw, come on," the mouthy teen said. "Do 'Grandma Got Run Over By A Reindeer'."

"Shut up," said the woman in the fleece top, snapping her head around to stare down the boy.

Ah, at last, some quiet, I thought. And no Christmas carols. What now? I drew in a breath. I surveyed the group. Country. Yes, country. An idea came.

Almost heaven. I strummed and sang looking around the room. *West Virginia.* Good thus far. *Blue Ridge Mountains, Shenandoah River.* I heard a female voice join in and then another. *Dark and dusky painted in the sky. Misty taste of moonshine, teardrop in my eye...* We got through the verse to the chorus. *Take me home, country roads, to the place I belong; West Virginia, mountain mama take me home, down country roads.* There was silence when I finished.

And then a familiar voice spoke. The mouthy teen boy said in a small, hushed voice, "That's where momma's goin'. She's goin' down a country road to heaven."

This was New York, not West Virginia, but he got it. I could hear some muffled crying in the background, but not from him. He remained transfixed by his discovery, not moving a muscle or saying anything more. His eyes looked off in space; maybe he was imagining his mother in heaven.

I wasn't aware that Chris and the social worker were making passes by this room during my stay, monitoring the situation, and ready to pounce if anything disruptive occurred. Unruly behavior wasn't common at the House. Later they told me they leaned up against the wall by the door, out of sight, listening when things quieted down.

"How did you do that?"

"I didn't. The music did."

~~

For family members coping with the illness of a loved one, or trying to understand a seemingly senseless tragedy, people of all ages and all backgrounds have experienced music's power to soothe, heal and bolster their courage in difficult times.

Joan Scott Lowe, BSN, LMT, CMP

Vibrations, Vol. 11, #2

Newsletter of the American Institute of Holistic Theology

Chapter 5

Finding My Musical Niche

Darby Music Shop was my toy store. While my mother's fingers walked through bins and bookshelves of sheet music, theory workbooks, and graded piano books for her piano students, I cruised the aisles of the cramped shop, stopping to study the musical instruments displayed on velvet-covered shelves in long lighted glass cases, or hanging on side walls like precious works of art in a small museum. I cannot recall exactly how old I was when this fascination began. But I cannot recall a time when I wasn't smitten with musical instruments.

I imagined myself playing each one: woody clarinets, glistening trumpets, silver flutes, all manner of drums. I longed to handle them, try them out, hear their sounds. My sights always came to rest on the long wall of beautiful wooden stringed instruments: violins, violas, guitars, their elegant, exotic shapes and warm brown and tan hues creating a rich, textured tapestry. Mom often finished her business long before I was ready to leave the store and whisked me away from that magical world in the music store. She didn't see—or she ignored—the gleam in my eyes.

At age six I eagerly began piano lessons with my mother. She gave up on me after only a few sessions. We locked horns. At the time I didn't understand why she became angry with me: I thought I was pleasing her with my ability to imitate what she would play for me. She insisted I read the music.

"Just play it for me, Mama," I would beg.

At first she did, and I would play the song back to her, looking down at my little stubby child's fingers reaching for the proper notes on the keyboard. Once she determined I wasn't going to look at the music, she ceased pre-playing songs for me in hopes I would resort to the printed pages in my Little Oxford Piano Course. Her plan failed, and she refused to continue my lessons.

Only as an adult did I understand that her music degree in voice and piano taught her only to read music and teach others to do so as well. She didn't know what to do with me. In her eyes I was being disobedient. I thought I was a failure, but I still experimented on the piano, playing music by heart and making up my own songs. My mother was not at all interested in my approach to making music.

After a couple of years, many trips to Darby Music, and a lot of pleading, I was finally allowed to take home one of the violins off the music store wall. I was eight years old. I would have been delighted with any instrument, but the size and fit mattered. The crusty, ancient store clerk with pince-nez glasses, a wrinkled white shirt rolled up at the sleeves, and billowy pants held up by bulging suspenders, measured my hands and arms. His eyes scanned the violin wall until he pointed to the one right for me. It shone with a deep orange-brown finish, slick ebony fingerboard, rounded tuning pegs, and chin rest. As he placed it on my shoulder, I could smell fresh varnish and see no scratches on its finish, a sign that it was a brand new instrument, not someone else's cast-off. My parents made it clear that they would only rent this violin by the month, citing my unwillingness to cooperate with piano lessons.

I devoured violin books, happy to learn to read music as well as play by ear under the tutelage of Mr. Belfiglio, a passionate Italian maestro, who came once a week to my house to give me lessons. Within months I was invited to join the advanced orchestra at school and moved my way up to first violin. The joy of the orchestral music, its harmony, its textures, its challenges, and also the fun with all the other music students and their instruments, drew me further into the love of music. Since memorization came so naturally, performing solos, duets, and in ensembles didn't faze me in the least.

Despite my thrill with violin-playing, I remained intrigued by the guitars at Darby Music. How could you play all those strings? Six, sometimes twelve? The guitar produced so many varied sounds and, unlike the violin, could be both a solo and accompanying instrument, the latter an ally for my singing voice.

I was a teen, still playing violin, when our family moved away from the school district with the orchestra, away from beloved Mr. Belfiglio and my music friends, to northern Virginia, where there was no strings program in the schools. Playing solos was not my preference, but I gave in when the band teacher asked me to play in the high school's Christmas concert. I remember standing up in front of an audience of new friends and their families in the school auditorium playing "O Holy Night" on my violin, accompanied by the choral director on piano. Kids stared, asked where I learned to play. Some didn't even know what instrument I was playing. I felt awkward, freakish.

Peter, Paul and Mary, Ian and Sylvia, Bob Dylan, and Joan Baez flooded the airwaves in 1964. Folk music fueled my desire to play guitar. My boyfriend let me borrow his father's old Gibson F-hole steel-stringed guitar for two weeks; another friend taught me my first four chords, G, Em, Am, D7. I practiced every spare minute, my fingertips burning with pain as I pressed them into the old, taut rusted strings of the antique Gibson. At night I crouched, guitar in hand, in my walk-in closet, door closed, defying my bedtime, playing and singing after lights out. *Where have all the flowers gone, long time passing?* G, Em, Am, D7; G, Em, Am, D7, over and over. My first song.

When the two weeks of the borrowed guitar deal ended, a few school friends and I piled into a large gas-guzzling sedan and sped to Arlington's National Pawn Shop, where they sold nylon-stringed guitars for twenty-five dollars (I'd heard that nylon strings didn't eat away at your fingertips like steel strings). I had saved just enough babysitting money to buy the guitar and contribute to a quarter-tank of gas.

I knew nothing about guitars but was thrilled to have my own. It looked okay and played pretty well too. Exactly three weeks after its purchase, I accompanied myself and two girlfriends in the high school Hootenanny. We won first place and took home twenty-five dollars each with our arrangement of "Where Have All the Flowers Gone?" in three-part harmony, my arrangement, all improvised.

That guitar accompanied me to the College of William and Mary, where I joined the Down County Four, a folk-rock group that performed all over campus and the surrounding Williamsburg area. We used no printed music, but made up our own vocal and instrumental arrangements after listening to the vinyl records we played in the listening room of the campus center. I played guitar and sang for singalongs in the dorm and gave guitar lessons in trade for typing my English papers. I volunteered at Eastern State, the regional mental hospital, playing and singing for groups of blank-faced patients seated in dimly lit, sparsely furnished rooms. I was frightened in that place, but when I saw a smile emerge from the darkness or heard a lone voice sing along with me, my discomfort vanished. I toted my guitar across the tracks to the segregated primary school and entertained the kids in a third-grade class where I lent a hand once a week. Their faces lit up with the music. They clapped, sang, even danced, encircling me, feeling my soft long hair, patting my light skin. Their responses remained close to me as I crossed back over the tracks and returned to the insular world of a college coed.

As my skills improved, I recognized the limitations of a twenty-five-dollar guitar: I needed a better instrument. During semester break I drove to Alexandria Music Store, knowing its reputation for fine instruments. My excitement and fascination for music stores had not waned, and I was itching to get into that magic place. Another wall of beautifully displayed guitars met my eyes. I locked on to one in particular, medium-sized, classical-style, with a warm honey-toned finish. At eighteen, I didn't need permission to take the instrument off the wall and play it. This little beauty melted against my chest, nestled perfectly into my left hand. I wrapped my right arm around its body and began to play and sing. *Hush a bye, don't you cry, go to sleep ye little baby.* Celestial, mellow, moving. I'd found a soulmate. This was the one, a hand-made Swedish Goya guitar.

But—one hundred eighty-nine dollars, plus tax, on sale. And the holiday price expired in two days. I cashed in my savings bonds and robbed my scanty bank account. That still wasn't enough so I brokered a loan with my mother—not an easy task—but she gave in, even though she didn't think much of my musical pursuits. She made it clear I was expected to pay back every penny.

Nevertheless, the Goya was mine!

~~

Fast forward forty-five years. Still bursting with music, I unpack and tune that same Goya guitar, my precious musical companion, and head down the hallway at Mountain Valley Hospice House as a Certified Music Practitioner. My Martin and Yamaha steel-string guitars usually remain at home, since the Goya's sweet tones complement the hushed, even holy atmosphere of the House. The glinty, outspoken sound of steel strings is too big for frail, often overwhelmed patients in small rooms.

By this time I have come to fully appreciate my abilities to memorize, play by ear, and improvise both vocally and instrumentally. Other musicians, including my mother, envy these skills. I wonder if they can be taught. Are they skills or gifts? In the therapeutic setting, having no musical scores propped on a music stand between me and my patients allows me to maintain an intimate connection with them, to readily observe subtle changes as the music progresses, and to make immediate adjustments. The music becomes seamless since I don't need to stop and shuffle sheets of music or turn pages in a book. Live, personal, one-on-one bedside music blossoms into relationship at a deep unspoken level, an ideal healing environment in which to use my unbridled gifts.

Let It Be Wild

Formal education builds a beautiful gilded cage around a mysterious gift. Here, it says, these are the ways to employ your love of music. You must learn this method and that theory. You must hold your hands this way and memorize great artists' compositions. If you dare to create something new, it must include these things and be in this form in order to be received by people who can judge greatness.

What if it is possible to turn the cage inside out, to use it merely as a ribcage to cradle the musical heart that came into the world to re-create the songs that gave it life, in its own perfect pitch, in its own perfect way?

The artist who asks these questions becomes one who can bring all his own experiences and gifts to his instrument (and voice) with no plans, no pages, no doubt.

—Kathy Godfrey, "Let It Be Wild"
WNC Woman, June 2012
used by permission

Chapter 6

"I Never Saw a Wolf"

Len's door was still closed, as it had been every time I came to the House. I asked about him. The nurses explained he was so medically compromised that he refused to spend any time with a stranger, fearing the embarrassment of having an accident. I inwardly cringed. No wonder this poor man isolated himself. I wanted badly to give him music. He probably needed it. I caught a glimpse of him later that day as he sat, door ajar, in his room, huddled up under several blankets, watching an old movie on a television with the volume turned off. I just waved at him and moved on, knowing that if I was to offer him music, I would need to proceed slowly.

I could tell my guitar caught his eye. He didn't wave back, but followed the Goya as I passed. I learned on my next visit that he asked a nurse about me after I left. He told her he heard my music and cracked his door open himself in an effort to listen to the songs better.

When I saw him again he was walking at a slow pace in the patient wing of the House, dragging his oxygen tank behind him. He was a skeleton of a man. His eyes and his skin were yellow. I introduced myself and asked if he might like some music later. He hesitated and finally said,

his own instrument along with the promise for lessons.

"I'll make sure you get a letter from Hospice for your donation. You can take it off your taxes." Dad seemed uninterested in the offer.

"And thank you. A lot. Len will be surprised. I'll let you know how it goes."

Dad just smiled.

I called the House from my car and related the great news about the guitar. The secretary couldn't believe the good fortune. She put down the receiver to share the news with staff. "I'll call the local newspaper for photos and a story. We'll have ice cream and cake. Everyone can come." Even a date was set for the event.

As I drove home, my only regret was that Len wasn't with me at the music store. I imagined that his intrigue with all the instruments, at least the guitars, matched mine. Everything had happened so fast. I would have loved seeing Len's expression when Dad removed a guitar from the wall peg and handed it to him.

Then Len became very ill. His door remained closed once again. I prayed and held my breath. I decided to bring the guitar and all its accoutrements with me to the House, maybe shed some hope on the situation by having them nearby. After showing them to the staff, I stowed them in a closet near the nurses' station, next to Len's room. We exchanged the same worried looks, wondering silently if Len would ever see the guitar.

Two weeks later, we rejoiced when he beat the odds. His door opened and we set a new date for the guitar presentation. Newspaper reporters and photographers arrived, the volunteer coordinator carried a cake decorated with a guitar, nurses and administration gathered in the hall outside Len's open door. I held the guitar, still in its case. We entered slowly. Len looked up surprised and perplexed by the crowd in his room.

"Hi, Len. I've got something for you. Do you know what this is?" Our excitement mounted.

"Yeah, I think it's a guitar."

I opened the case, removed the precious instrument, and held it up to him. "Yes, and it's yours."

I placed the instrument in his hands. Cameras flashed, applause broke out, the nurses cried, and Len sat expressionless, still unbelieving.

"I have books and a music stand, a guitar stand, and big picks. And I promise to teach you how to play. How does that sound?"

There was no response. Finally, he spoke quietly, rather overcome, looking down. "That sounds good. Thanks."

He would not let go of that guitar, not to eat or drink the party treats, not to leave his chair, not for anything. He held that instrument like a baby, close to his chest, studying the strings, the shiny tuning pegs, the gorgeous wood finish. I left him and the festivities for a while to tend other patients but stopped back by his room so we could talk about his upcoming lessons. He was still cradling that guitar, lost in his new possession, smiling easily.

"Clip the nails on your left hand for a lesson next week," I said. "Maybe a nurse can help you. Then try to press on the strings with those fingertips once in a while. You can start building up calluses that way." I showed him how to hold the pick and strum lightly. He was in heaven.

"See you in a week."

The next week Len was not in his room. Then I smelled cigarette smoke and saw his door to the outdoor patio cracked, his oxygen rig left inside beside his lounge chair. A volunteer sat with him, a requirement for going outside the House. Zipped up in a camouflage jacket, his head topped with a matching baseball cap, he sat at the patio table looking out into the winter woods, deeply inhaling a smoke, one of the habits that had brought on his illness and landed him at the House.

Len noticed I had come into his room. He nodded. His new guitar sat in its stand very close to his lounge chair. His picks and music rested on the tray of the silver music stand awaiting his first music lesson. I tuned up both our guitars and awaited his slow entry back inside. He kept his camo jacket on, as he often did, and lowered himself into his lounger. I unfolded my portable chair next to him, sat down, then placed his guitar in a good position for his thin body and small hands to envelop it as he played. He shivered. Was it a chill from the outdoors, a bit of fear, or excitement? His droopy eyes brightened. He was ready. I paged through the beginner's book to find the description of guitar parts. Body, sound hole, fret, neck, first string, second string, I explained, pointing to each part of his guitar.

"Let's try a chord," I suggested. "At the third fret," and I counted up the guitar neck for him, "wrap your thumb around the top string, the thick one, the one closest to you. Now press your ring finger on the third fret of the bottom string." I counted up again and placed his delicate finger on the string. "Hold these fingers tight against those two strings and strum across all of them with your pick. This is the easy way to play a G."

He caressed that big pick and tentatively pulled it across the strings, hearing his first chord. It was muddled and unmusical, but it was as pleasing as any Johnny Cash music to this lonely, deprived man. He strummed again and again and smiled. I added the D7 chord, calling it another easy chord in that lesson and wrote out a diagram of both chords on a notebook page. As I was pointing out the chord diagrams in his music book, I saw him squint and lean closer to the page. Was he unable to see it? I pulled the music stand closer. Or, my heart stopped, could he read?

Our next lesson didn't turn out the way I planned. Nor did the next or the next. He couldn't play the easy G or D7. I felt like a failure. I shouldn't have called them easy chords. Had I done harm to this fragile man? I adapted the lessons so no reading was required, not daring to push too hard to determine his literacy. I had him play only single notes, not chords, in hopes of stringing together a melody of his choice.

Len was a proud man despite his limitations. He was trying to please me. I wanted him to please himself. His fingertips were tender and sore from pressing the strings against the fret board, and his concentration came and went in waves like his nausea, fatigue, and depression. It was just too much.

I thought back to my private music studio where I had taught guitar and dulcimer lessons for years, and I reflected on how many students with disabilities seemed to gravitate toward me: learning disabled, ADHD, seizure-disordered, autistic, Tourette's, wheelchair-bound. But I had never taught a dying person.

Len seemed happy, relieved for me to play his guitar and sing to him as he rested in his chair, buried under his animal print blankets, focusing on my fingers as they moved around the strings. We never officially ended the lessons; instead we left a "someday when you feel better" hanging out there in his limited future. I came to understand that merely having the guitar next to him, all golden and shiny new, having his own possession to look at, to make him feel like he was in a different place, satisfied a longing Len may have harbored all his tattered life.

Len's door remained open most days. I entered freely. He became talkative in between songs. He told me stories of his cross-country trips in his rig, seeing cacti, buttes, the desert, orange rock formations, vast sunsets; hauling across the Rockies in ice and snow, unsure if he would make it, then rolling down the mountains back to flat land and searing one-hundred-degree heat. He saw roadrunners, snakes, mountain goats, coyotes, but he never saw a wolf, he said, turning his head to gaze outside at the snowy, evergreen-treed hill a short distance from his Hospice window. I think at that moment he was hoping to see a wolf lift its head to the sky and howl a long, mournful song for him. His comments led me to reach around to my music bag. I slid my Native American flute out of its sack and began to play. He continued to look out the window, lost in the music.

"There's a wolf out there," I said. He nodded, smiled. I continued. Low, easy, slow. Haunting tones, and far away. Note into note in a minor mode. And then I ended.

"Can ya play that wolf song again?"

He was transformed. I was with him. We were out in the wilderness, moonlight illuminating a gray wolf, its face to the sky, serenading the night. I glanced at Len's blanket. The wolf on his coverlet had come alive for both of us.

"I think there's a female out there too, with pups in the den. Let's see if I can coax them out with some faster music."

He beamed and watched the hill as I filled his room with lighter notes, dancing and playing like the tiny furballs who emerged from their hiding place. "Do you see them?"

"Yeah." He couldn't avert his eyes. "Play some more so they stay out there."

I played the flute and the wolves continued to appear for weeks on end. A poster of a wolf showed up on his wall. He wore a new cap with a wolf on it. A new wolf blanket wrapped him up warm. I learned that Mike, another Hospice volunteer, collaborated with our wolf stories, bringing Len these wolf-themed gifts.

When spring arrived, Mike took Len fishing. Pictures of this adventure, Len in a lawn chair trying to cast a line out, with Mike holding him securely so he didn't fall forward into the lake, took their place next to the wolf on Len's wall. And then a family picture of Len's father and mother together with a war medal and a locket, was hung next to the other pictures in a beautiful shadow box on the wall near Len's window.

Len had acquired a new family, a home, people who loved and cared for him. A reason to live. And live he did, outlasting the admitting doctor's initial sentence of three months, tops.

Len asked me to a party he was throwing. What? Len, a party? It was his birthday and he had ordered shrimp, steaks, salad, fruit, and potatoes for a feast out on the Hospice patio. He said he wanted to spend every cent of his Social Security check for this celebration. All the staff came, along with other able patients and Mike and me. We ordered a cake and blew up balloons to complete the event. Mike and I played music together on that sunny April mountain day—he was a harmonica player. Folks danced and sang along. Len sat back observing, pleased with his party, his birthday gift for us.

For over a year Len lived the high life at Hospice. He even sent out Christmas cards with a return address for the first time in his life. I placed mine in a safe place. And then Len's door remained closed more often, and I knew his illness was finally taking him away. I never really knew what his diagnosis was.

It was devastating to lose patients, especially the long-term ones. He was like family. I so earnestly wanted to play music for him, but his pride would not allow anyone but the nurses and Mike into his room; Mike, a man, a brother, familiar with Len's ailments. I wondered, though, if Len was protecting me from seeing him in his dying state. He was like that. I sent messages of love through the door via Mike and the nurses.

Then one day Len's door was wide open. And he was gone. The guitar sat by his chair.

I took the instrument and walked to the Serenity Room at the end of the patient hall, where I stood it in its shiny stand next to the piano near the windows. I stepped back to enjoy the beauty of the instrument in the morning light. A heavy sense of loss came over me as I walked back to the nurses' station to get my instruments and prepare to go to other patients.

I inhaled deeply. God help me do this work.

~~

The next time I was at the House I went directly to the Serenity Room to see if a guitar hanger had been installed on the wall. Seeing it in place, I took Len's guitar and slid the neck into the padded holder. Then I took a framed newspaper article with the photo of Len holding his new guitar and hung it on the wall next to the treasured instrument.

Other guitars in holders now lined the wall, too. Touched by the story in the local newspaper about Len's dream and Dad's generosity, folks donated their usable guitars to the House. Len's now joined their ranks.

Later that day, I saw a man carry Len's guitar into the room of a newly admitted patient. He noticed I was watching him. "Mom wants me to sing some hymns for her," he said. "Is it okay to use this guitar?"

"Yes," I said. "Len would be so pleased."

Music is God's gift to man, the only art of Heaven given to earth, the only art of earth we take to Heaven.

—Walter Savage Landor

Chapter 7

Musical Morphine

Kimberley, a young woman in her forties, reduced to skin and bones, lay either in her bed or in her recliner with as few sheets or blankets as possible on her tender skin. The slightest movement of her rigid body, even the most gentle touch from a nurse or a family member, induced enough pain that she cried out. The morphine was not working as well as the Hospice staff hoped. She hardly slept.

"I have my lap harp with me today. I think it might help her relax. What do you think?" I asked the charge nurse.

"She's in too much pain for anything right now. I don't think it's a good idea."

"I could play outside her room in the hallway."

"Okay. But we'll check on her."

I unfolded my small black, portable chair, uncased my harp, and sat down outside Kimberley's door. I could see her from my position in the hall, but I could not measure her reactions up close, as I needed to. A furrowed brow, restless hands and feet, a frown, a clenched jaw, even the tiniest tic under the chin. These signs told me to either stop or change the music, but I could not see them. So I just played: soft arpeggios, minor chords, slowly, easily, with a steady beat, one type of music for intense pain. A nurse passed me and poked her head in the door to check on Kimberley.

"Where's the music coming from?" I overheard.

"Our therapeutic musician's outside your door."

"Can she come in? I want to hear it better."

I entered her room and settled myself at the side of Kimberley's bed and began again. The taut skin stretched over her skeletal hands cracked and bled, her gnarled fingers were nearly frozen. Her face was tight, pulled back like a plastic surgery job gone bad. I could see her legs, stiff and angled, beneath the single sheet. A box-like aluminum rack on top of her mattress prevented the sheet from touching her tangled feet. These were only the visible ravishes of scleroderma.

"Hi, Kimberley, I'm Robin, the House musician. I'm here to offer you soft, soothing music. If you feel like going to sleep please do so, and if you've had enough music give me a sign and I'll stop. This is for you. I'm not a performer, I'm another member of the Hospice team. I hope this will give you some pleasure, some peace. Thank you for inviting me in."

She nodded slowly, eyeing the maple harp with its warm, natural finish.

I started playing again, this time an Irish air, "Southwind," with its sweeping chords and luscious melody. The fluid nature of the harp and its vibrational qualities often reach into the human body far beyond other instruments—to deep hurting places, to a patient's physical and emotional pain. The harp's ministering timbre is associated with ascendance into a spiritual place, a healing place, heaven. Within minutes I saw Kimberley's claw-like fingers release and relax a bit onto her bedcovers. And then her eyes fluttered as she whispered.

"I haven't ever heard anything like this before. I haven't felt like this before."

She fell into a deep, lovely sleep. I continued to play Irish airs, my flowing hands sending music and love to her pained, crooked ones, to her entire body. She breathed more deeply, sighing with the exhales. I crept out of the room, pulled the door to, and left her fast asleep.

The harp became her requested instrument; we laughingly called it her "sleeping pill." She was quite adamant about my entering her room and playing music under any circumstance, despite the nurses' assessments some days that she was in too much agony to be disturbed. Soon the staff, seeing the miraculous effects of the musical intervention, embraced my music for Kimberley. They nicknamed me the "Musical Morphine."

Something unusual about Kimberley stuck with me long after she succumbed to her awful illness. Her smile through excruciating pain, her gratitude, her bright spirit filled her Hospice room with a permeating glow. She didn't complain or whine. Her mood remained upbeat and positive. How could this woman maintain her graciousness in all that pain? Was that temperament a gift? Or was it learned over a long decline in health? With that attitude, she naturally attracted staff and family to her. We all sought to give our best to this amazing woman.

~~

I carried that little harp to many a room in Hospice. Its celestial overtones soothed anxious souls. Mary, an elderly woman with signs of dementia, enjoyed visits from her large, attentive family. I didn't choose to interrupt these visits so I passed by her room on several occasions when they were present. One afternoon when she was alone, I entered. She lay in her bed, clutching a plush tan teddy bear, wide-eyed and rather confused about who I was. I greeted her and slowly recited my spiel about offering her music. She allowed me in. Noticing a well-read, open Bible on her bed stand, I began to play music with a religious spin. I sang the melody and words accompanying myself with the harp. *Amazing grace, how sweet the sound.* She perked up. I sang two verses, then changed songs.

I come to the garden alone while the dew is still on the roses.

She spoke. "I know that," she said, raising her arms with the teddy still held tightly. "This is my baby. I have to take care of him."

I nodded. "Does he have a name?"

She stared blankly. I continued. *And He walks with me and He talks with me, and He tells me I am His own.* She began to sing, then stopped herself. "I can't sing anymore." I encouraged her to try again. She remained silent.

"What's that?" she asked pointing to the harp.

"It's a small lap harp. Do you want me to play more music?"

She moved her head in agreement. I alternated between sacred and secular music, harp alone, then with vocals. She fell asleep with her teddy resting on her cheek. I left quietly and moved down the hall.

During my next visit to Mary's room a nurse entered with an amused expression on her face. "Mary's family came shortly after you left last week and Mary told them a woman with a harp was in her room. They freaked out. You know, woman, harp, dying mother. They thought this was the end coming for good ol' mom." The nurse and I laughed out loud together, but I learned a bit of a lesson. From then on I left a business card on patients' tray tables to authenticate any reports of a harp-playing woman in their rooms.

I made a point to meet Mary's family, let them see that I was a live harpist, and we all chuckled about the harp story. "Yep, we thought she was goin' on outta here. She talks about you whenever we come. The music is very special to her. She used to sing a lot. She's a Methodist."

The next thing I knew I was being invited to perform for Mary's ninetieth birthday. The whole family would attend, it would be a surprise, and they wanted some music, family favorites. They insisted on paying me since I would be making a separate trip as a private performer for this occasion. From my home on the lake to Hospice was a good fifty or more miles round-trip, so I accepted the offer.

The party was a hit. Mary was alert, talkative, even funny. "What a party for an old woman," she said. I blew out all the stops with a complete program of multiple instruments—guitar, Appalachian dulcimer, harmonica, harp, bowed psaltery, and of course, the limberjack, minus his Christmas outfit. We closed the door to Mary's room since the entire gang, including Mary, sang along. *I come from Alabama with a banjo on my knee*, then *Daisy, Daisy give me your answer true*. And finally, the Happy Birthday song.

Everyone knew this was probably Mary's last birthday, but the mood remained festive, buoyant. Her delight in her family, the cake, a dozen roses, plus her cards, gifts, and the music were infectious. No tears for this woman. I performed way beyond my agreed time and was taken aback when the oldest son handed me a check for double the amount we had brokered. I began to speak. He waved me off, shaking his head. "You really are an angel. Take it."

~~

There were days when I encountered a light load at the House. Patients were sleeping or meeting with the House chaplain or social worker. Out-of-town guests often visited, crowding around their loved one's bed. I noticed how many were making small talk, fussing with the bed covers, getting a glass of water, doing anything to distract their charged emotional reactions from the reality of death in front of them. How well I understood the difficulty of seeing a lifelong friend or a family member in this situation. Sometimes, while playing for a patient, I flashed back to my dad dying under Hospice care. Folks felt awkward, helpless under these circumstances. I thanked my lucky stars that I had something to offer, to give, to do when I entered a Hospice room. My music delivered two gifts in one—a gift for the listener and the other for me, all wrapped up together in the same beautiful package.

On slow days at the House I parked myself in the hallway outside the doors of the administrative staff. Their work, like mine, wasn't easy. Since the House held only eight beds for patients, the administrators became very involved in day-to-day events in their lives. Patients' needs were urgent, sometimes critical, and above all the highest priority of the House. Comfort, dignity, peace were the hallmarks of Hospice care, so the staff scrambled to maintain these high standards at all times. And after all was said and done, no matter how hard we tried, every single one of our patients slipped away from us. I attempted to ease our grief with quiet, flowing harp music, unobtrusive, heartfelt, uninterrupted. Whatever moved me, whatever came forth out of that instrument, came from a place deep inside myself.

Maybe I was an angel: maybe this is what an angel is, and does: heal, and bring peace.

"How did you know we needed that really badly today?" asked Julie, the receptionist and intake counselor. Her eyes were glazed over with tears as she came out of her office to give me a hug. "I think I'm in heaven," she said.

"I hope you are."

Even if you are not a singer by nature or talent, you are not left out. If you have a voice, it is your birthright to celebrate life with song.

—"Harmonizing with the Universe"

Daily OM, Dec. 9, 2010

Chapter 8

Kurt Flies Away

Kurt sang like a choirboy. Neither his tall, burly physique nor his career as a state trooper matched—or prepared me for—his voice, a sweet, high tenor harmonizing from memory. When he sang, his blue eyes sparkled and his gruffness melted away like ice on a sunny day. He was retired now, and in poor health. I met him at church and encouraged him to join the choir. We were members now for two years at the small white clapboard New England-style Presbyterian Church. Its wide red open double doors welcomed new choir members along with anyone else who entered the cozy sanctuary.

"I can't read music," Kurt said, apologizing for not accepting my invitation to Tuesday choir practice.

"Just show up and try it. I can help you."

Sure enough he walked right up to the choir loft, his cane tapping the wooden steps, ready for rehearsal on the following Tuesday at four p.m.

"What do I need?" He was more forthright than I imagined.

My mother, the choir director, scrambled to assemble music into a black folder, then passed him the packet along with a list of music for the month, handwritten on notebook paper in her somewhat illegible script. She was eighty years old at the time. Kurt was seventy-five, but his multiple heart operations had aged him.

Thus began a love affair over music between me and Kurt. When he became discouraged over the difficulty of the choir music, I calmed him down, helped him find his notes. His natural ability to harmonize, singing his own made-up music high above the melody, actually prevailed over the written notes most of the time, but no one cared. My mother told him, "Kurt, just do what you do."—a real stretch for her. But she knew his presence and his beautiful voice lent a special ambiance to the front of the church where he sat with the choir each Sunday morning.

Kurt approached me one July morning after church, carrying a bulging manila folder. He opened it to show me his collection of favorite hymns, gospel tunes, folk songs, the copies now dog-eared and yellowing.

"My mother and I sang these together. I stood next to her as she played the piano, and I think that's where I learned to sing harmony. I go back to these copies for the words."

Besides church choir and working toward my CMP, another outlet for my musical energy was forming a music committee within the local arts network. Its reputation had plummeted along with its bank account when the former president resigned under suspicious circumstances. When New York City folks migrated north in the summer to their camps on the lake, I seized this opportunity to begin a concert series featuring affordable professional musicians along with an open mic opportunity in the Village Park on Sunday afternoons. I hoped the well-heeled summer people along with the local folk might bring picnics and lawn chairs and toss in a few bucks when we passed the hat during intermission.

"Would you sing with me at open mic?" Kurt eyed me for a reaction. "I've never sung in public, except in church, but I think I can do it if you sing with me," he said.

"Sure. What do you have in mind?" I said, rather surprised at his request and my quick response.

"'Precious Memories'. And maybe 'I'll Fly Away'."

"I love those songs. Great choices. We'll need to rehearse. When are you free?"

Kurt's wife drove him out to my lake house a couple of times a week until we felt secure in the music. I played guitar and sang melody. He sang his signature harmony. We practiced the songs over and over, more for his confidence than for his musicality.

Our turn on Sunday afternoon at open mic arrived. We sang late in the program. Kurt was nervous, sweating, and out of breath. I worried about the performance placing too much strain on his fragile heart.

Lots of church members plus his family sat in the audience, knowing what a big day this was for him. When our act was announced, my husband jumped up out of his lawn chair in the front row to help Kurt as he wobbled up the rickety stage stairs, using his cane to steady himself. I followed, and we stepped into place on the stage before the microphones. He looked at me, his expression asking, "Do you think I can do this?" I nodded with a grin and began the guitar intro. His nerves settled down once he began singing, his liquid tenor soaring above my melody. *Precious mem'ries, unseen angels, sent from somewhere to my soul; how they linger, ever near me, and the sacred scenes unfold.*

He sang his best and really wowed the crowd, then easily slid into our next number. *Some bright morning when this life is o'er, I'll fly away. To a home on God's celestial shore, I'll fly away.* The lyrics rattled me a bit. I wondered if they affected him. Did he know he was singing his own farewell with these words? When the applause broke out, I stepped back from the mic and watched him in his glory. He was glowing, center stage, soaking up the attention.

After this success, Kurt's desire to perform at open mic amplified, but his health declined. He never did sing a solo, but through the summer open mics with me by his side, he overcame any shyness he had about singing in public.

By the fall his dwindling breath and energy from his inoperable heart condition finally robbed him of his singing voice. He was unable to navigate the steps up to the choir loft and, with regret, handed in his black choir folder and dropped out of choir. The cardiologist said Kurt's heart could give out any day.

But Kurt had one last request.

"I'd like to sing 'I'll Fly Away' with you and Heidi in church. Maybe three-part harmony. She already agreed, if you will."

Heidi was his youngest daughter, his only blood child. He and his wife had adopted three children after giving up on having their own. Then Heidi, the little miracle baby, appeared. Kurt held a special affection for his blonde, blue-eyed girl.

"Of course I will. I'll let Mom know so she can add us to next month's choir roster. I think we can be ready by then." I didn't want to delay too long. Kurt was noticeably failing.

Heidi, Kurt, and I practiced our three parts. Sometimes he became so winded that he had to sit to sing, but we pressed on, his determination overcoming his infirmity.

On our appointed Sunday we positioned ourselves in the front pew. Kurt's wife sat next to him holding a small tape recorder. We didn't attempt to scale the choir loft stairs, but stood on the floor. Kurt's complexion by now was pasty, colorless due to lack of oxygen, but he was eager to get this appearance in. We held our breath as he pushed himself up to stand and face the congregation. He was beaming. We began singing after my brief guitar lead-in. *Some bright morning when this life is o'er, I'll fly away...*

There were those words again. I felt sure Kurt knew exactly what he was singing this time.

We saw congregants wiping their eyes. Then they clapped and sang. Kurt's great harmonies, his triumph, brought a standing ovation, despite the church's policy about not erupting with applause in a worship service. No one fussed about it on this occasion. This joy was straight from heaven.

~~

As Kurt's heart slowed, he descended into total dependence on his tiny wife, who could barely assist him at home by herself. She called me to come over and talk with them about Hospice.

Kurt was admitted to the House a few days later. Our music migrated to his room next to the nurses' station, where he sat in a recliner, singing with me once again, with the aid of oxygen flowing freely into his lungs through a long, clear plastic tube. He had brought his manila folder of favorite songs and requested we sing one after the other, until I suggested he take a rest: he would have sung himself sick unless I stopped our sessions. I know the music distracted him, gave him hope in the darkness of his dying, lifted his spirits away from the irregular beating of his heart. Over the weeks we tore through that folder of music and then tackled an old red hymnal from church. He sang on.

And then he couldn't.

I entered his room on a bright winter day, ready to sing. He sat as usual in his recliner and welcomed me. I could see his eyes drooping with fatigue. His hands didn't reach for his music folder or the red hymnal on his chair-side table. His breathing had changed; now it was labored and staggering.

"I can't sing today," he said, huffing out those words as if he had run a marathon. Tears glazed over his weary eyes. I took a deep breath to keep my emotions in check.

"I'll sing for you, if you want. You can put your head back and listen this time."

"Okay," he said, choking on that one word.

After I sang just two songs, he said he was tired and wanted to take a nap. He looked away from me, down at the floor. I think he couldn't bear having the music fill his ears without being able to join in as he always had. By now we were a duo, music buddies, close friends. He had found a voice he never knew he had.

With this new development, I hated telling him I was heading south in a couple of days, escaping the winter weather for a few weeks. I finally bent over his recliner and hugged him for a long time, kissed his cheek, then mentioned my trip. He looked up. Our eyes met. I stood motionless, unable to say good-bye. So instead I said I'd stay in touch, then collected my guitar, walked toward the door and turned back toward him. "I love you, Kurt," I said, waving, hurrying out the door. Once I was in the hallway and out of Kurt's earshot, I covered my face, leaned forward against the wall, and cried out the grief that I had dammed up in my throat for a long time.

While I was in the South, I called Kurt's wife and daughter on a regular basis, keeping abreast of his condition. When they contacted me, I knew why they were calling.

Kurt died peacefully. They tried to choose a date for his memorial service so I could participate, but the extended family was unable to accommodate that time frame. I mourned not being present.

I am told that the church was packed for his service. The choir sang and lots of people got up to tell stories about big, burly Kurt.

But what really stuck in everyone's mind was the final music. A small tape recorder played a recording of Kurt, Heidi, and me singing "I'll Fly Away."

I'll Fly Away

Albert E. Brumley

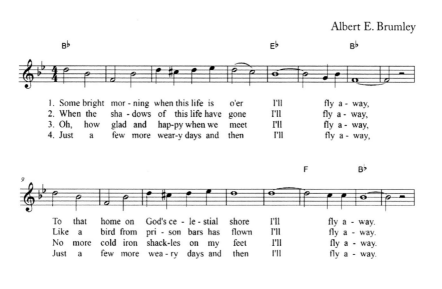

1. Some bright mor - ning when this life is o'er I'll fly a - way,
2. When the sha - dows of this life have gone I'll fly a - way,
3. Oh, how glad and hap-py when we meet I'll fly a - way,
4. Just a few more wear-y days and then I'll fly a - way,

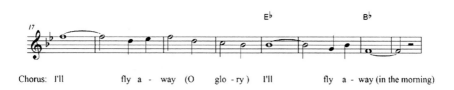

To that home on God's ce - le - stial shore I'll fly a - way.
Like a bird from pri - son bars has flown I'll fly a - way.
No more cold iron shack-les on my feet I'll fly a - way.
Just a few more wea - ry days and then I'll fly a - way.

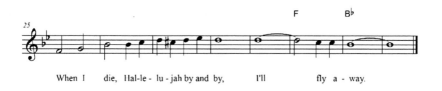

Chorus: I'll fly a - way (O glo - ry) I'll fly a - way (in the morning)

When I die, Hal-le - lu - jah by and by, I'll fly a - way.

Chapter 9

Dealer's Choice

The phone rang. It startled me: I was deep into reading my email. Sun reflecting off the frozen lake had warmed me into a stupor.

"Hello?" I answered.

"Is this Robin Gaiser?"

"Yes, it is."

"This is Linda Rains from Nathan Littauer Hospital Extended Care. I think you've been here a couple of times playing and singing for one of our patients, Mr. Duncan."

I panicked. "Yes, I have. He's my cousin. I hope that was okay."

"Oh, yeah. I'd like to know if you'd come here as a part-time employee doing the same thing you did for your cousin."

"I'm not finished my internship. So I'm not certified. I'm at Hospice House and I'll be done in about three weeks. And I'm not a music therapist, I'm a music practitioner. It's different. They've got four-year degrees and we've got—"

She cut me off.

"What's your fee? We pay hourly for part-time."

I didn't want to sound dumb, but I'd never considered a fee. I hadn't received my graduation certificate or my official badge. I knew what the New York City folks got, fifty dollars an hour, but I certainly wasn't in the city. I was in rural upstate New York. One Certified Music Practitioner I knew from rural New Hampshire told me she got $30 an hour. "The range is between thirty and fifty an hour but I understand if—"

"We'll pay you fifty an hour but we can only afford four hours a month. Is that okay? When can you start?"

"Uh, yeah. When do you want me?" I almost told her I had to wait until I was officially certified, but she spoke before I had time to say another word.

"By the time you complete the background check and fingerprinting and get the physical and shots, it'll be close to when you graduate. This place is really slow. I'll email you the names of the people you need to call to set those up. Call me if you have any problems. I'll call you when I get all your paperwork. Any questions?"

"I'm sorry, but can you give me your name again? And your telephone number? And who will I be working under?"

"Me. Linda Rains. I run the Recreation Department for Extended Care. My phone is—"

This time I cut her off. "Thanks, but I'm not a performer, not a recreation musician. I'm trained to do live bedside music for—"

She interrupted again. "I just talked to your supervisor at Hospice. He told me what you do. Give me your email."

I rattled off my computer address to her, rather dazed and befuddled. "I'll be in touch. Bye."

I had hardly gotten a word in edgewise, but I was out of breath. What had I just done? I knew very little about the facility or Linda. When I sang for my dying cousin at Extended Care I merely marched straight to his room and back out again. I did notice the halls were long and the rooms were cramped. And when I sang and played, patients in wheelchairs gathered outside his open door.

~~

I completed my internship at Hospice but agreed to stay on as a volunteer. They would pay my gas mileage and subsidize the workshops and enrichment classes I needed to maintain my certification. My thoughts about payment for my music services vacillated between wanting to earn money and wanting to freely give. Experiences at Hospice made me realize my work was more a ministry than a job. Kimberley and Bob, Len, Dolores and Kurt ... these were not numbers or names on a chart or a greaseboard. These were beautiful people with a story and a life and a dying wish.

I was moving away from my old self, the one who negotiated payment for music rendered. Those music contracts kept me separated from my inmost desires, to reach people with music, to heal, to honor, to bless. I was ready to leave the realm of a professional waltzing in to do her music on a time clock and then breezing out, payment in hand, to move on to the next job. This was not like that. That was not me anymore. Payment or not, I had to do this work.

The balance between Hospice and my actual job at the hospital required juggling time and energy. The leisurely pace at Hospice, with its short, hushed eight-bed hallway of patients, gave way to a noisy, chaotic atmosphere of eighty-eight beds, mostly filled. Televisions—company for lonely old folks—blared non-stop, monitors beeped menacing emergencies, nurses and assistants rushed in and out of patients' rooms, cleaning crews with loud whining machines polished linoleum floors. Worst of all was the continuous mournful, frightened crying out from patients. "Help me, help me. Help me! Will someone help me?" Someone was always crying, "Help me."

How could I help all these people? Where would I start? Four wings, eighty-eight beds. And four paid hours a month.

The Recreation Department office was overstuffed with craft materials—felt, sequins, magic markers, pipe cleaners, colored paper, crayons, coloring books. Board games and plush animals, books, comics, playing cards, and puzzles teetered on sagging wall shelves. A cart with afternoon treats sat in the middle of the only walking space in the room. Desks were deep in paperwork. There was no place to put my instrument case or my coat. This job, like my music, was going to require improvisation.

Linda Rains, an ample-bodied woman with long dark brown hair, a round face, and a huge smile, found her way through the maze of stuff to the copy machine and made me a copy of a list of patients' names and their room numbers. I wondered if her continual smile was her coping mechanism for getting through the day in this environment. She laid the paper down on top of a pile of newspapers and starred the names of the most needy patients with a big purple pen, topped with pink feathers, which she unearthed from under a heap of birthday wrapping paper. I folded the list and a blank piece of paper into my pocket along with my own simple pen. Then I jammed my harmonica into my other pocket next to my business cards, looped the lanyard bearing my new badge and hospital ID over my neck, grabbed my guitar and portable chair, and entered the first wing.

Wheelchairs with people slumped forward, drooling and dozing, lined the hallway. A man raised his head as I passed him. "Oh, that a guitar? You gonna play it?"

Why not, I thought. So I opened up my chair and sat down right there in the middle of the hall and began playing and singing. *Way down upon the Swannee River, far, far away, there's where my heart is yearnin' ever, there's where the old folks stay.* Other heads lifted, empty eyes gawked at me. Some of the blank stares yielded to signs of recognition as the music began to wake up drugged and fuzzy brains. "Sing along with me," I said. *Daisy, Daisy, give me your answer true. I'm half-crazy all for the love of you.* Then right into *East Side, West Side, all around the town.* I heard some weak attempts at singing. And a smile or two broke out on a couple of tired, wrinkled faces. I could just stay here all afternoon, I thought. But there was a list in my pocket with stars by the names of the patients most in need ... yet how could anyone be more needy than these folks here in this hallway?

I soon found out.

Emanating from the room where I was planning to offer music was the harsh voice of a woman yelling out, "Get the hell in here. Will someone take care o' me?" When Helen's name was starred, Linda warned me she cussed a blue streak. I entered gingerly. Helen mistook me for a nurse. "Fix my sweater, goddamn it. I'm hot. You always take so long to get in here." Helen's late stage Chronic Obstructive Pulmonary Disorder left her bedridden, tethered to oxygen full time. And very grumpy. Her breathing was rapid, frantic; she was fitful and restless. She finally wrestled herself out of her sweater. This small gesture left her exhausted, sweating profusely, and heaving for breath. She noticed me. "Who are you?" she blurted out in between gasps for air.

I introduced myself and asked her if she wanted some music. "I suppose so," she exhaled. "Why not." She took in another breath. "There's nothin' else to do in this damn place."

She inhaled again. I remembered the information about the entrainment principle, that a person's heartbeat and respiration will naturally match, or entrain, to the beat of music. I began at a breakneck pace, one which matched Helen's breathing rate. *Rock-a my soul in the bosom of Abraham, rock-a my soul in the bosom of Abraham, rock-a my soul in the bosom of Abraham, oh, rock-a my soul.* I kept that beat up and then began ever so gradually to reduce the tempo, watching Helen's chest, listening to her breathing, occasionally glancing at the heart monitor. Her inhalations and exhalations began to slow, her heart rate began to match my rhythm. I brought the tempo down some more. She stayed with me, and then I maintained a rhythm in the high-normal range of seventy heartbeats per minute. I have no idea how much time this took, but her chest stopped heaving and she settled down.

"Are you a nurse?"

"No. I'm the new musician for Extended Care patients."

She cocked her head and said, "Well, you can stay here all afternoon."

"Do you have any favorite music? Or shall I just give you dealer's choice?" She looked like a woman who might have played some poker in her day. And a woman who definitely smoked like a stack. She didn't wear the hospital-issue nightgown but donned a flimsy green number over a lace bra. There were no pictures of family around her room, and her fingernails were painted a bright red.

"Dealer's choice," she said, winking.

I had struck a chord.

Frankie and Johnny were lovers. Oh, lordy, how they could love. They tried to be true to each other. Just as true as the stars above. He was her man. But he done her wrong. I accompanied myself using a snappy, jazzy style where I slapped the side of my guitar as I played the chords. Pretty soon I noticed those red fingernails tap, tap, tapping out the rhythm, her tired head swaying back and forth in time.

I played a few more familiar tunes and glanced at my watch. I was planning to get in two hours of music today, cover an entire hallway, and already over a half hour was gone.

"Don't quit on me," she begged. I think Frankie and Johnny's story prompted this way of asking me not to leave her. I imagined she had been done wrong by a few Johnnies over the years.

"I promise to come back." I was bothered by the fact that my return to Helen's room might take a month or more. I had to make the rounds to so many other starred names on my list.

"How 'bout one more?" I asked. I was already growing fond of this woman. *Amazing grace, how sweet the sound, that saved a soul like me. I once was lost but now I'm found, was blind but now I see.* Tears formed in the corners of her eyes and she put her head back onto her pillow. That hard face softened as she listened to all four verses. I repeated the first verse a cappella, then eased the volume down with a nice decrescendo. She fell asleep.

Whenever I worked the halls at Extended Care I made a point to serenade Helen more often than the others. With advanced COPD, she could be expected to expire any day. But she proved to be a tough cookie and outlived my prognosis. When she finally began to decline, she was often sleeping soundly, breathing heavily, when I stuck my head in her door. She had told me to wake her when I found her like that, but I chose not to disturb the peacefulness she enjoyed with the assistance of regular morphine injections. Finally her heart stopped, and she died in her sleep.

I never got to say a final good-bye, but I consoled myself with the remembrance of the many good-byes we said to each other every time I departed her room, never knowing whether this was the last one. As I thought about our acquaintance I realized how little I knew about her. She kept it that way, and it was not my place to pry.

She always asked about my family. I showed her pictures of our grown children, and told her about their lives. When our first grandchild arrived, she celebrated him as if he were her own. "Do you have any pictures of the baby?" I handed her a thick envelope of photos. She studied each one for a long time while I sang to her. "He's so beautiful. Make sure you sing to him," she said looking up with a loving smile.

When I passed her empty room, I lowered my head, said a short blessing, and let the tears fall. Then I counted back, wondering how long I had sung and played for her.

It had been just shy of two years.

Only those who will risk going too far can possibly find out how far one can go.

—T. S. Eliot

Chapter 10

"One, Two, Three Strikes You're Out"

Some days my work at Extended Care didn't go the way I anticipated. As I made my way to the recreation office to leave my instrument cases and coat, I noticed a strikingly handsome elderly gentleman seated outside his room in a wheelchair. He was stylishly dressed in cords and a sweater, gray hair expertly combed, expensive shoes shined to a gloss, clear eyes the color of a bluebird. I had not seen him before so I reasoned he was a new patient. His name was posted on the wall outside his room. John. I took note.

"Hi, John," I said to him as I walked by, knowing I would return shortly to offer him music.

No one was around the recreation office so I edged sideways through the usual maze, unpacked my instruments, looked for patient lists on Linda's desk and, finding none, navigated my way back out of the office to the hall where John sat. I wondered if his name was starred on any list.

I was aware that new patients often benefited from music as they adjusted to life in unfamiliar surroundings. The loss of health was difficult enough, but when a patient was finally placed in a care facility, the loss of home, family, friends, pets, and freedom often begat confusion, withdrawal, depression, or anger. Music soothes, orients, relaxes a person in such situations. Obviously someone on the outside was ensuring John was meticulously tended: very few patients looked the way he did. I would add my music services to this man's care in his new home.

I introduced myself, asked if he wanted music. Those blue eyes stared through me. He didn't answer, but he maintained a pleasant expression on his face. I parked my little chair near him, sat down and began to play and sing. It was summer, we were in New York, and the Yankees were winning. I hoped he was a fan. *Take me out to the ball game, take me out with the crowd.* His eyes remained fixed on me. *Buy me some peanuts and cracker jacks, I don't care if I ever get back.* He was really hard to read. No signs of recognition. *So it's root, root, root for the home team, if they don't win it's a shame.* Surely he'll react to the next phrase. Everyone does. *For it's one, two, three strikes you're out at the old ballgame.*

"John, did you like that?" No response at all except a little shuffling of his feet. Maybe he needed some calm, restful music. I changed the mood, played a classical arpeggio on my Goya as an introduction to "Peace Is Flowing Like a River." I often chose this song for its steady, easy beat, its low pitch, its message of peace and love and healing. He scowled. This was not working.

Before I could change gears, he hollered, "Get out of here! Get out!" Suddenly he jerked his long arm from his lap and took a powerful swing at me. I pulled back just in time, barely avoiding the full brunt of his large hand on my face. I looked around to see if anyone had seen this outburst. No one. Stunned, I scooted my chair farther away from him, stood up, and inhaled deeply, backing away, trying to regain my composure. What had happened? What did I do wrong? Did I do harm? And then I began to tremble all over. A nurse appeared in the hallway.

"That man there, John," I pointed, wide-eyed. "He just tried to hit me."

"Did he get you?" she asked.

"No, I ducked in time."

"Didn't anyone warn you he's Alzheimers and he's violent? You have to keep your distance. That's why he's here. Wife couldn't manage him."

"Oh," I replied, still shaking.

She walked on.

This was a first. I turned to walk slowly back to the recreation office, replaying the incident in my mind, hearing the angry shouts to get out, reliving the sudden attempt to attack me. I glared back at him still sitting in his wheelchair, his face emotionless, his beautiful blue eyes staring straight ahead, oblivious. He was ill, but in that moment I hated him. He made me feel like a failure. And for the first time I was afraid.

I stopped, still shaking all over. Was this my fault?

I wanted to go home, forget this work. It was too hard. Too risky. How many others would reject me? Take a swing at me? And why didn't anyone tell me?

I entered the office and retreated to a corner. I had to sit down, recover. I needed to talk to someone—but no one was in the office. I felt myself begin to cry, then hoped no one would enter and see me like this. An assistant entered. She spotted me. I wiped my eyes and told her the story. She came across the room, opened her arms and hugged me.

"That happens to me, too."

"How can you take it?"

"I just talk about it and finally I'm over it. There was one patient I refused to help since he was so violent. We got the male nurses to handle him."

"Thanks. Can you tell me if there are any other violent ones?"

"No. Only John."

It takes strength to bear well what we cannot change.

—Joan Chittester, *The Gift of Years*

Chapter 11

Music: 1, Meds: 0

"Are there any special needs today?" I caught a floor nurse's attention as she hustled down the hallway. The nurses were always in a hurry.

"Yeah, Bonnie, 34 B, east. Dying. Struggling. A lot of pain," she said, still in motion.

Asking a nurse this question had become my strategy for zeroing in on the most needy patients at Extended Care. The patient list was not kept up to date, and more often than not when I arrived no one was in the recreation office to star the list or direct me to the rooms of those folks I ought to see.

Eighty-eight patients, four wings, and four hours a month had begun to disturb me. I was driven to respond to every one of those pitiful cries that met me when I opened the doors to my workplace. *Help me, help me,* rang in my ears long after I packed up my instruments and departed the facility for the day. Even my favorite CDs during the long drive back to my lake house could not block out the chorus of urgent voices.

Bonnie shared a cramped room with a woman seated in a wheelchair, mesmerized by a blaring TV whose volume overwhelmed the dark, suffocating space. A skimpy curtain separated the two patients as if it were meant to offer privacy and quiet.

"Would you be willing to lower the sound on your TV while I play some music for Bonnie?" I asked the roommate.

The woman glared at me, but then fumbled for her remote and reduced the volume a little.

"Thanks," I said, wishing she had turned the sound completely off.

My heart stopped when I stepped into Bonnie's side of the curtain. She lay on a narrow hospital bed, curled in a fetal position, naked except for an adult diaper. Not even a sheet covered her emaciated body. As I approached I could hear her moaning above the sickly music of the afternoon soap opera still whining from her roommate's television. A middle-aged woman with short uncombed hair sat slumped in a chair pushed back into the corner of the oppressive room. The air smelled thick, warm, putrid.

"She's in terrible pain. She's scared. It hurts to touch her. I'm a friend."

"Maybe I can help," I said, moving closer to Bonnie. "Hi, Bonnie, I've brought a small harp. Let's see if the music can relax you a bit. I'll watch carefully to see if it's too much." I shortened the usual entry protocol. There was no time for that.

She looked up at me through glassy, desperate eyes.

I placed my chair next to her bed and began playing slow arrhythmic music in a low, minor key, one note at a time. The research I studied in my classes told me that since her breathing was labored and her pain and anxiety levels high, this music, without a beat or recognizable melody, would work best to calm her, ease her intense pain. The last thing I wanted to do was tax her heart or her neurological system with complex, beating, or stimulating sounds. After about ten minutes of continual playing, I observed that her hands slightly opened, her clenched jaw flexed.

I played on.

Then her breathing deepened and became more rhythmic. Her moaning eventually gave way to sighing. I changed my tempo to match her respirations and felt myself begin to breathe along with her, our chests rising and falling together, synchronized in perfect harmony. My breath, the music, was filling her dying body and soul with all the healing power I could muster. Her eyelids dropped as she sighed more easily, more quietly with every exhale.

The music was working. I could feel the heavy air dissipate in the room. I sensed movement in the corner where the friend was seated, noticed her weary head tilt forward into her raised hands. Who knows how long this woman had kept a vigil at Bonnie's bedside.

I continued playing. Bonnie settled into a restful state, moving her body carefully out of the fetal position and on to her back. Her arms rested now at her sides. To my surprise the entire space on both sides of the curtain was suddenly hushed, except for the sound of my music. The TV noise had actually ceased. I wondered if Bonnie's roommate had also surrendered to the vibrating strings of my therapeutic harp. The tranquility allowed me to relax, let go of some of the intensity required to tend this dying woman. I pulled back, exhaling a silent prayer of gratitude, still offering soft, unobtrusive music with a slow beat. At times I hummed along.

Then I heard it.

Bonnie jerked awake from her reverie. Her friend's head snapped with a fright. A nursing assistant burst into the room pushing a rickety upright vitals machine, its wheels clackety-clacking against the hard vinyl floor and broadcast in a loud, commanding voice, "Bonnie, time to take your blood pressure and temp."

I immediately stopped playing and moved myself out of the way to make room for the equipment and the nurse.

Then it hit me.

"The music just calmed her down. Does this have to be done right now?" I asked respectfully, holding back my incipient anger.

"Doctor's orders. Hospital policy," she said with authority, wrapping the blood pressure cuff roughly around Bonnie's upper arm. Bonnie cringed, cried out as the nurse pumped the cuff which squeezed relentlessly against what was left of a skeletal extremity. Bonnie tightened her face muscles; her brow furrowed, tears ran from her eyes. Then the nurse stuck a thermometer in between parched, paper-thin lips. Bonnie gagged, nearly wretched.

I had to look away.

The nurse left pushing the rattling machine. I repositioned myself near Bonnie and strummed my fingers slowly up and down the harp strings, attempting to restore the calmness and quiet that had once engulfed the room.

Then as abruptly as she exited, the nurse returned waving an injection needle.

"She's due for a morphine shot," she announced, again in a loud voice. "Bonnie, can you roll over so I can get your hip?"

I wanted to cry. Roll over? A shot? Why not a dropper in the side of her mouth?

Bonnie wailed as the nurse nudged her over on her side to expose what was left of a hip. The needle entered loose skin, near a protruding bone. Bonnie jumped, let out a high pitched scream as the needle pierced her side.

The nurse's medically required interventions left Bonnie in a frightening state. Anxiety, pain, fear strangled her body and mind once again. Her eyes were wild. The space I had laboriously created with music was now destroyed, frantic. I began playing, knowing that the morphine would take up to a quarter of an hour before it had any effect. Fifteen minutes passed. Bonnie remained agitated, her hands clenched, her jaw set, her face wrenched up in agony. More time passed with no change.

The morphine dose must have been inadequate. Bonnie moaned with every irregular breath. Her friend wept, and I played on without success. Then, adding to the mayhem, I heard the TV start up once again, a newscaster's urgent voice squawking through the fake wall between my dying Bonnie and her clueless roommate. I marshalled all my skills to replace this nightmare with serenity. I struggled to keep my concentration on Bonnie and drown out the angry dialogue rising up in my head. I wanted to yell across the curtain. But I knew the roommate was not the whole problem.

I finally gave up, exhausted. Resting my harp against my chair I stood. Leaning over Bonnie's bed, my arms raised, palms open, I sang a blessing. This was all I had left to offer. *Go now in peace. Go now in peace. May the God of love surround you. Everywhere, everywhere you may go.* I think this blessing was for both of us.

"God bless you, Bonnie," I said softly, lingering next to her bedside for a while after the music ended.

I finally gathered up my chair and harp and exited. I had failed. Everything about Bonnie's care had failed.

On my way down the hall, I spotted the nursing assistant.

"Bonnie's still in terrible pain," I called to her as she entered another patient's room.

"She's not due for meds for another four hours," she replied, cocking her head out the doorway before she disappeared.

"But—" I called back. Then stopped.

There was no use.

From the introduction to Being Mortal
by Atul Gawande

You don't have to spend much time with the elderly or those with terminal illness to see how often medicine fails the people it is supposed to help. The waning days of our lives are given over to treatments that addle our brains and sap our bodies for a sliver's chance of benefit. They are spent in institutions—nursing homes and intensive care units—where regimented, anonymous routines cut us off from all the things that matter to us in life.

Our reluctance to honestly examine the experience of aging and dying has increased the harm we inflict on people and denied them the basic comforts they most need. Lacking a coherent view of how people might live successfully all the way to their very end, we have allowed our fates to be controlled by the imperatives of medicine, technology, and strangers.

Atul Gawande, *Being Mortal*
Metropolitan Books (Henry Holt & Company)
used by permission

Chapter 12

Parking My Ego

Why I do this work? Sometimes I wonder. As I recall story after story, I relive the searing impressions that these encounters with these people and their circumstances, some in the last days or hours of their lives, have imprinted on me. The very act of offering music to strangers who are navigating doorways into the unknown requires my intuition, my senses, my knowledge to absorb every subtle nuance of the individual men and women and their surroundings. I must be wide open. My eyes, my ears, my nose tell me something, crucial facts, but my soul, my psyche, my spirit often lead me to the deeper meaning of the situations. Why do I keep coming back?

The stock answer is about giving, meeting a great need, being useful and valued, making a contribution. But I could do that without exposing myself to the Johns and the Bonnies and the others whose lives, and whose dying, are described in this book. There are so many stories.

Another easy answer is that my early religious instruction told me to serve those in need, the lesser, the ill, the lonely, the hungry—and to use my gifts in doing so, or I would lose them. As a child I sat smitten at the feet of visiting missionaries who came to Wednesday night church potlucks and told heartrending stories. How could I ignore the photos of African children my age, big-eyed and puffed up with hungry bellies, covered with fly-infested sores on their naked bodies, staring out at me. My sense of the less fortunate was aroused at an early age.

While others give money, feed the hungry, work in shelters, build homes, join the Peace Corps, I make music. Not simply because I can, because it's what I do, but because music reaches into a restless, hungry place within me. I am coming to understand why at a visceral level.

So why music?

I see my great-grandfather's tarnished, ornate silver trombone resting in the arms of a wall display in my great room. He breathed music through this instrument before he passed it on to my grandfather, who then gave it to my father. They all played it. Across the room his ancient clarinet hides in a flaking wooden box fastened by a delicate clasp on top of a cabinet.

On a high shelf, my great-great-grandmother's zither asks me to play "Nearer My God to Thee" on its rusty strings, as she did most Sunday evenings for the family after supper. Small, sepia-toned hymnals that they held in their hands grace the shelves of a handmade, glass-front cabinet, a family heirloom, standing against another wall.

My maternal great-grandfather's ebony conductor's baton rises proudly out of an earthen vase, next to a photo of him in concert playing his violin decorated with a Beethoven head scroll enunciated with diamond eyes. I was supposed to inherit that violin, too, but no one knows how it disappeared.

My mother's chromatic harmonica from music school spews dried, filmy reeds next to a banjolin and a ukelin high on another shelf. The harmonica was new when I found it. My mother never played it, but I blew my first tune through it when I was nine. I am the one who used up the reeds.

On a long wall under the music shelves hang my guitars, violin, dulcimers. The harp, bowed psaltery, and Native American flutes sit atop my grandmother's hope chest, and autoharps, hammer dulcimer, and harmonicas in many keys—silent but ready to burst forth with song—await me in my music closet.

~~

My earliest music memory takes me to my grandparents' parlor where the ancient, dark oak upright piano, its top weighed down with sheet music, books, and hymnals, beckons my mother's hands to play it. I am less than three, sitting on my mother's lap. She is playing and singing from the children's music books she takes to the elementary school for her students. *I had a little nut tree, nothing would it bear, but a silver nutmeg and a golden pear. The merry-go-round, goes toodle-ee-ooh, come take a ride there's a pony for you.* And of course, *Twinkle, twinkle, little star, how I wonder what you are.* I easily sing these songs from memory today. I have recorded them for my children and grandchildren. Those children's music books line my shelves, a gift from my mother. This music must be kept alive.

My father strokes my forehead, singing me to sleep. *Bye, baby bunting, Daddy's gone a hunting. Gone to get a rabbit skin to wrap his baby Robin in.* I snuggle my slumber pup, feel safe, loved, warm. He sings when our family takes car trips. We join him. When he sings we are happy, calm, unafraid. His moods, his actions are predictable. He just drives and sings, and I feel joy. We are the family I long to have.

~~

My grandfather opens the blue hymnal, we stand to sing, he holds my hand during the service at the Northville United Methodist Church. I am visiting for two weeks of summer vacation. *Fairest Lord Jesus, ruler of all nature, Son of God and Son of Man.* I am nine. I can sing the alto harmony with his tenor. My grandmother holds my other hand and sings the melody. I delight in our trio.

Later I sit at the ancient piano and play tunes for them by heart. They hover nearby and listen.

"How can you do that?" My grandfather asks as he smiles down at me. I feel cherished.

How can I do that, I ask myself? Play songs from memory, play anything I hear. Make up songs to suit the occasion. Improvise. The music emanates from some mysterious place. That's what I do. That's the gift. And connection, safety, love, comfort, joy, fill me, take the music to my depths as they did so long ago. They are embedded. When I play and sing for others, I release these feelings for them, and for myself. I give. We all receive.

I am playing the church organ for Bible School. I am thrilled. I can play every song without music. Mrs. Curry and Doris Main nod at me with pleasure as I sit in the choir loft, my ponytails tied with red ribbons, swinging rhythmically as I reach for the notes on the high console. They take me under their wing as their own. I think they know how hard I try to please them and my family, especially my musical mother.

~~

Music is where I feel loved. Past, present. Music is where I give love. Why do I continue to enter rooms of strangers who are suffering, dying, cursing, diminished, unwashed? Because of love. I don't see hollow faces, blank stares, decaying bodies. I see the faces of God in these human beings. Precious people with stories, contributions, presence. Music pays tribute to their lives, often coaxes out their life stories, gives them worth, but most of all loves them when they are lost, weak, vulnerable.

"I want to die."

"Why doesn't God take me?"

"Why am I still alive?"

"I want to go home."

"I'm useless."

You are my sunshine, my only sunshine; you make me happy when skies are gray; you'll never know dear how much I love you, please don't take my sunshine away. A ray of hope, purpose, life enters the gloomy space. Love fills the room. How can I turn my back on the needs, the helplessness, the pain? I can sing to the cries of "Help me, help me." And when I do I am singing to my own dark nights when I cry out for someone to help me. I have music. I am loved.

Tell me why the stars do shine, tell me why the ivy twines, tell me why the sky's so blue, and I will tell you, just why I love you. Because God made the stars to shine, because God made the ivy twine, because God made the skies so blue. Because God made you, that's why I love you.

Because God made you, that's why I love you. The dreary room fills with light. I want to feel needed. So I tend the needy. I want love, so I give love. I honor, bless, heal; and I am honored, blessed, healed. This is how it works. I don't fail when it doesn't work. I am not God, but God is always present. God is in charge. God lights the halo of love I envision encircling the patients' doors as I enter. I must keep these thoughts close to my heart lest my ego attempt to perform for my own glory.

~~

I am deeply aware of, and need to share, the grace, the energy, the gift I have been given. But I am only human. Between sessions, I must take a break, breathe deeply, and above all pray that my music brings healing in the highest sense of the word.

I do this now and I go forward.

I am a healer.

There is no greater and more living resonator of sound than the human body. Sound has an effect on each atom of the body, for each atom resounds.

—Hazrath Inayat Kahn

Chapter 13

Holding the Music in Her Hands

I am back at work at Extended Care. As usual I ask the nurses about serious needs. Lillian's name bursts forth from both nurses I approach in the hallway.

"She's ninety-six. Lonely. Sad. The only one left of her family and friends. Been with us for six years," said one nurse.

"Yeah, Lillian. She could use some company, cheering up. A sweet old soul. You'll love her," the other nurse chimed in.

Lillian's room was hushed, darkened by the curtains pulled tightly across the window. A hospital bed with the rails up rested in the middle of the private room. The television picture was on, but the sound was off. *Ahhh*, I thought, *no battling the noise.*

Bedcovers were heaped on the bed and I almost didn't discern that someone was buried beneath the tussle of blankets, sheets, and pillows. What I finally saw was a tiny head of flyaway gray hair, a puckered face the color of pancakes, and, as I got closer, two slits for eyes, oozing some thick, milky fluid. She saw me through the gooey eyes and raised her arms out of the bedcovers as if to greet me. She glanced at my harp then frantically pointed her crooked index fingers to her ears and tossed her head back and forth on her pillow.

What's she doing? I wondered and stood there to study her. Maybe she's saying she doesn't want music. Her motions continued. Then I caught on. She's telling me she can't hear. Why on earth did the nurses send me, a musician, to play and sing for a woman who is deaf? At first I was annoyed. I was probably the company they referred to, the warm body, the hand to hold. I can do that. Just sit there and be present. But that's not what I came to do. I smiled at Lillian as all these thoughts went through my head, nodding that I comprehended.

I unfolded my portable chair and sat as close to her as I could, up near her ear, playing my harp on its lowest strings where vibration is most intense. I had learned in classes that the body is seventy-five percent fluid and that vibration of that fluid is the way we experience sound. I also knew that the vagus nerve, located behind the ears, is the only nerve with connections to every organ in the body. I worked on those low strings, plucking extra hard for both volume and vibration. She still pointed to her ears, shaking her head that she could not hear the music. She frowned. I was in a quandary. I could not leave this lonely, isolated woman. But what would I do?

I had an idea.

~~

I was back in a school in Fairfax County, Virginia as a music educator. I had performed a program called "Music Soup" to a large group of elementary children dotting the gymnasium floor, when the principal approached me.

"That was great. Did you see how even our non-English-speaking children joined in? And I wonder if you have time to come down the hall to our classroom of special needs kids," she said.

"I have about a half hour before I need to leave to pick up my children from preschool. Yes, I can do that." I gathered up my guitar and harmonica and followed her down the cavernous, yellow-tiled hallway, wondering as I walked just what kind of children she meant.

She opened the door and before me was an assembly of maybe twelve children, nearly all in wheelchairs, some strapped in, others randomly waving their hands or rocking, and some completely inanimate, their heads hanging down toward their bellies. These kids were severely disabled.

She announced out loud to the group that I would be playing and singing music for them. I watched to see if anyone responded to her introduction. No one moved or changed expression.

I stood at the front of the class, feeling helpless, and began strumming my guitar and singing "Oh, Susannah" to no response—so I sang louder.

How is it that we think we need to raise our voices for disabled persons or for those who do not understand our language? My increased volume made no difference.

A pudgy, pinkish girl in the second row caught my eye. She was seated sideways in her chair. Her ears stuck out from her blonde curly hair and as I got closer, I noticed scales on her blue eyes. She had the look of an albino child.

"Patty's blind and deaf," I heard an adult voice say. It was one of the aides.

"Can I take her hands?" I asked.

"Yes, that's what she responds to."

I knelt on the floor next to her, up close so she could reach my guitar. I carefully took her hands and placed them flat against the body of the guitar and began strumming. She shivered, a funny little movement that seemed like excitement, and then I saw the brightest grin spread across her face. When I stopped playing, she tapped on the guitar as if to say "More, more." So I continued with the strumming, just chords with no singing. She smiled and shivered all the while. I hated to stop but there were others.

A boy sat to her left. He wore a bib, and was restrained by a soiled padded belt at his waist, keeping him from pitching forward in his wheelchair. His dark hair was greasy and uncombed, and I could see the bulge of a diaper in his gray sweatpants. No one commented about his condition, so I tried singing and playing for him. He didn't change his expression or show any response to the music. I put the guitar down on the floor next to me, kneeled near him and took out my harmonica. I placed the harmonica so it just touched his face, next to his ear, and began playing. His head came up slowly and he smiled. Then I heard attempts at vocalizations. He was trying to sing. Actually, he was singing. His kind of singing. And to me, at that moment, nothing could have sounded more beautiful.

I tried to serenade each student individually, but my half hour sped by quickly. "I have to go now," I said rather apologetically. "When I come to this school again I'll allow more time."

"Thank you. That was amazing. I can't get over the responses," said the principal, the aides nodding in agreement. "We need more music for these children."

~~

My memory brought me back to Lillian. There she was in her bed, tiny, silent, still staring up at me, still pointing to her ears. And unable to hear the harp.

Remembering those children in the special needs classroom, I knew I would not abandon Lillian. I would employ the skills I had learned as a music educator and try my luck once again.

Pointing to the harp and my ear in response to Lillian's gestures, I indicated to her that I had a new idea. She acknowledged me, but pointed to her ears again, this time with a quizzical look on her face. I stood up, knelt one of my legs on my chair, steadied the other leg on the floor and bent toward her. She looked up at me with curiosity, but I didn't notice any hesitation. I positioned the small, five-pound harp on some pillows next to her, and held it with my right hand. She reached over to touch its soft curved body. With my left hand I took one of her crooked little hands and opened each finger, then wrapped one finger at a time around the base of the sounding board. I did the same with her other hand. She didn't resist. In fact, her face brightened, excited about what might happen next. Once her grip on the harp was secure, I freed my right hand to pluck out a slow familiar single-string melody, singing the words to myself. *Twinkle, twinkle, little star. How I wonder what you are. Up above the world so high, like a diamond in the sky.*

She cried out, "I can hear it. I can hear the music!" She held on tightly as I steadied the harp. I saw a toothless grin widen across her baby face. Tears fell from those filmy eyes. *Twinkle, twinkle, little star, How I wonder what you are.*

I stopped, lifted the harp away, watching her. She looked puzzled, raised her hands, palms open. I was certain she was asking why I ended the harp music. I pointed to my back, already breaking in that awkward position. I didn't want it to give out. I knew I carried adequate liability insurance if something happened, but that wasn't the issue.

I took a couple of deep back stretches and leaned over Lillian once again with my harp in hand. This time she placed her own fingers around the sounding board and I plucked out melody after melody. When I finished, she motioned that she wanted to kiss me, puckering up her tiny colorless lips. "You are my best Christmas present," she exclaimed in a loud voice. It was February, but I loved the message. It really was Christmas. I offered her the backs of my hands and she slobbered kisses all over them, holding them securely with one of her hands and patting them with the other. She wouldn't let go.

I finally wiggled my hands away from her in order to motion that I needed to go. But I made it clear I would return. She understood, and waved exuberantly. I blew her kisses. She blew her own kisses back.

Once outside her door, I washed my hands and then wiped my harp down with special disinfectant cloths I carried. I felt disloyal cleaning Lillian's kisses off my hands and swabbing her innocent fingers off my harp. But I wasn't willing to take any chances, so I followed universal precautions both before and after seeing her—or any patient. In this case, that included my instrument.

Lillian's story followed me home that day. I told my husband and two friends about her, but kept to HIPAA rules by not mentioning her real name or her location. They were all smitten, amazed by the events. "You ought to write about this."

"Maybe I will."

I mused about Lillian all week. What a joy to reach her! On my next visit to her I brought the harp, but I also tucked a compact Marine Band harmonica into my pocket. She saw me enter her room and threw up her hands, gesturing to come nearer. I walked over to her bedside, pulled the silver harmonica from my slacks' pocket and held it up so she could see it. She nodded. Then I leaned over her, as I had done with the disabled boy years ago, placed the harmonica on her cheekbone and across her ear and began to play. Her little hands reached up and covered my hands on the harmonica and she tapped out the rhythm of each tune perfectly. Skin against skin. My breath pushing musical notes, rhythmic vibration into her via her facial bones. *She'll be comin' round the mountain when she comes.* She didn't hear the music with her ears, but she felt it with her body. *I wish I was an apple a hangin' on a tree and every time my Cindy passed she'd take a bite of me.* She named every single song I played.

"I know that one. My teacher sang it. I went to Cranberry Creek, the one-room school, up to Benson. Not there anymore. Made it into a history building or something." She spoke at a full volume. Maybe she could hear her own voice that way. I'm sure the entire hallway did.

I acknowledged her story with a nod, looked her in the eye and wished I could tell her that it was my grandmother's idea to rescue the rotting school building and restore it as the historical society's museum in Northville. I wondered if she knew my grandmother, who was near Lillian's age, and still living. I took a chance and leaned in toward my tiny patient, gently pushing away the errant gray hairs sprouting from her ear. Cupping my hands, I spoke directly into her ear through my makeshift megaphone.

"Did you ever know Charlotte Duncan Russell?" I all but yelled, enunciating each syllable. She looked up at me with a pained expression and pointed to her ears, shaking her head in the same telltale "no." She truly could not hear with her ears. I felt badly for experimenting with her, so I pulled out the harmonica again, played more folk tunes, then followed with some harp music.

Whenever I played, her hands either rested on the harp or embraced my hands on the harmonica, but each maneuver involved touching, getting as close to me as she could. I wanted to take her face in my hands and caress her, thinking how patients were so tactilely deprived. The staff tried its best to rub backs, hold hands, comb hair, stroke foreheads, pat arms, and hug, but the demands on their time prevented much of that. Lillian was touched and held in so many ways through the music.

She insisted on kissing me after each session. She pointed to her cheek every time, motioning for me to kiss her there. But I blew kisses and offered my hands instead. She kissed the backs of my hands and blew kisses to me as I passed through her door. Then I washed down. This was our routine.

After I had been playing for Lillian for several weeks, I started my usual trek down the hall to her room. I met a nurse as I walked and mentioned in passing that I was going to Lillian's room. I didn't expect the response she gave me.

"Lillian passed away two days ago. Peaceful. Just died in her sleep. She's happy now. I heard about how you played the harp and harmonica for her so she could hear. That's such a miracle," she said.

I thanked her for her kind words. "Lillian was a dear. You know she knew every tune I played for her, but she couldn't hear one word I spoke." She smiled at me.

"We wondered if she really heard the music or if it was just a nice story. Lillian is the one who told us about it. You really did a lot for her. You made her very happy whether she heard the music or not." She moved on with that comment, disappearing into a patient's room.

I stood motionless in the hall, hugging my harp and fingering the harmonica in my pocket. A wave of guilt washed over me. I could have done more for Lillian. I knew Lillian had heard my music, but in this moment that didn't feel like enough.

I wished I had kissed her.

~~

After Lillian died a nurse told me that she had succumbed to a urinary tract infection, a common ailment among sedentary older folks. I learned she was on Comfort Care, Extended Care's version of Hospice, and I wondered if she had arranged that for herself. She demonstrated a sound enough mind to make that decision, and I didn't know of any designated healthcare proxy who was still alive to assist her. I recalled that there were no IV poles, monitors, feeding tubes in her room, and she didn't receive antibiotics: she was simply kept hydrated with water and comfortable with pain meds. And, thankfully, when I offered her music, there were no interruptions for taking her vitals.

Yet even though I knew she was happy and ready to die, I missed her. Selfishly, I wanted her back, wanted to feel those sloppy kisses on the backs of my hands again.

But the philosophy often espoused by Eastern thinkers, that death is a natural extension of life, was beginning to seep into my thoughts more often after patients like Lillian passed on. I could see that in this way, her life progressed to its natural outcome. As this new idea took root in my head and my heart, a strange feeling came over me: I was actually joyful about her death. Of course I missed her, grieved her loss. But we all die. And she died well.

~~

This is who I want to be in the world. This is who I think we are supposed to be, people who help call forth human beings from deep inside hopelessness.

—Anne Lamott

Stitches: A Handbook on Meaning, Hope, and Repair

Chapter 14

Semper Fi

I strolled past Lillian's empty room seeing a bare, stripped bed instead of a heap of covers burying my miniature friend. Remembering the musical surprise of her hearing music through vibration had often brought a smile to my face, but now I could also feel joy that she had died well and naturally.

My thoughts quickly changed gears as I strolled to my next patient, Ron, forty or so, depressed, at Extended Care for rehab. That's all I knew. He had a private room on the sunny side of the building. Warm light was streaming through his window. His door was ajar and he was resting on his bed, facing away from me. He wore long sweatpants, a gray T-shirt, and white athletic socks, the uniform of the day for physical and occupational therapy. I tapped gently on the door to see if he responded. He asked who was there.

"Hi, Ron. I'm Robin, the hospital musician. I'm wondering if you might like some restful, easy-going music this afternoon. You can just stay right where you are and fall asleep if you want."

"Naw, thanks, but I don't think I want it today." He rolled over on his back and turned his head to face me. I recognized the emblem on his shirt.

"You a Marine?" I asked, still keeping my distance, standing in his doorway. His attention snapped to with this question.

"Yes, Ma'am," he answered with the crisp, polite response the Corps taught its recruits.

"My dad was a Marine Colonel, pilot, World War II."

"Oh, yeah?" He shifted onto an elbow.

"The youngest Marine flyer in the war. Fifty-six combat missions before he turned twenty. Philippines. Shot down three times. Escaped."

There was a long pause, then Ron spoke quietly. "I was in Iraq. Don't like to talk about it." He lay back on his bed. I wondered if he was in rehab for Post-Traumatic Stress Disorder, since I didn't see any bandages, scars, or signs of disfigurement. Then I saw the wheelchair in the corner.

"Thank you for your service," I said. And then I don't know what came over me but I raised my guitar and began strumming chords and singing quietly despite his initial request for no music. *From the Halls of Montezuma, to the shores of Tripoli; we will fight our country's battle from the land and from the sea.* How well I knew "The Marine Hymn": given my father's lifelong dedication to the Corps, it was our family's national anthem. *First to fight for right and freedom and to keep our honor clean. We are proud to claim the title of United States Marines.*

I held the silence after my last chord, waiting to receive any clues about how the music affected him. He didn't speak. He didn't look at me, but stared at the ceiling.

"My first husband was killed in Vietnam," I said. "Second Lieutenant in Khe Sahn. 1968. He was twenty-two. Bad times." I don't know why I told him this. But I knew how Marines stuck together.

His eyes met mine as he raised his head. "I'm really sorry, Ma'am."

"Yeah, war's pretty nasty. But Marines are the best."

"Yes, Ma'am."

"Do you mind if I sing one more song to you?"

"No, Ma'am." His shoulders relaxed a bit and he lay back down on his bed.

God bless America, land that I love; stand beside her, and guide her with a light through the night from above.

I sang the entire song, pouring my heart out to this wounded man. I thought I detected him blinking tears from his eyes, but I chose not to look too hard. He was proud, a Marine. Marines didn't cry.

"Well, I'll pack up now," I said, feeling a little awkward. "And get going. I'll check in with you another day."

"Thanks, Ma'am." He kept his words and his emotions intact.

"Semper Fi," I said as I turned to leave, noticing the Marine Corps emblem taped above his name on the wall next to the door.

"Semper Fi," I heard back as I walked away, down the hall to my next patient.

~~

The next week I went to Ron's room. No Marine emblems on the wall, no wheelchair. I got an empty feeling.

Seeing a nurse in the hall I asked, "Where's Ron, the patient from this room?"

"He's not here anymore. Left last week."

"Where'd he go?"

"I think he went to Albany VA Hospital, but don't quote me. We never really know what happens to patients when they leave here," she said continuing down the hall.

"Thanks," I said, calling after her.

I stayed there a minute thinking how the VA hospital would be better equipped to handle both physical and emotional issues for a returning soldier, but I wondered if it offered therapeutic music. Ron seemed to relax, open up when I sang to him. And how ironic that I shared my own personal story with him. I hoped I hadn't crossed the line. Shaking my head I turned and moved on to check on a new patient.

I'd never know if I had done the right thing with my Marine friend.

~~

There is a deep and mysterious paradox here, for while such music makes one experience pain and grief more intensely, it brings solace and consolation at the same time.

—Oliver Sacks, *Musicophilia*

Chapter 15

Deathly Afraid

After so many days at Extended Care I chose to take a breather the next week and follow my heart to Hospice, the easier of the two locations for me, with fewer patients, less noise, no odors, and no intrusive medical procedures. I always looked forward to the peace and quiet I would find at Hospice when I eased myself inside the double doors, my musical instruments nestled in their black padded cases and slung over my back.

Winter was waning but ice covered the parking lot in dark, treacherous patches. Heaps of filthy plowed snow, leftovers from the first accumulation back in late October, still obscured the grass and the sidewalks. A lot of melting would take place on this sunny afternoon, one of those blue-sky gifts of the mountains. As I opened my car door and slid off the seat to stand, I felt an urge to fling out my arms and sing at the top of my lungs. *The hills are alive with the sounds of music* came to mind. I would even twirl like Julie Andrews in the opening scene of *The Sound of Music*, but I restrained myself since most of the administrative windows faced the parking lot.

I picked my way across the black ice to the doors, nudged them open with my knee, and let myself in.

Something was different.

Hospice took extra pains to guard patients and visitors from the sounds and sights of emergencies, but today I heard intermittent crying and then saw nurses and staff racing in and out of a patient's room near the medical desk midway down the hallway.

Kathleen spotted me and rushed forward. "Thank heaven. You've come at the right time. We've tried everything but she won't calm down."

"Who is it? What's up?" I asked as we walked down the hall toward the room with all the commotion.

I had never seen Kathleen so frazzled.

"Peggy was admitted yesterday and then took a quick turn this morning. Her pain level spiked, her meds aren't working, and she's terrified. She may be actively dying. We ordered stronger meds but they aren't here yet. Everything happened so fast."

I stashed my instrument cases and coat, then stopped myself from going directly to this patient's room. I stood still. I needed to think about the information from classes on music for persons in the active dying state. I remembered being surprised that even the Hospice nurses in my class thought familiar music would be the right choice: movie and Broadway tunes, hymns, 1940s and '50s hits, the patient's favorite music if we knew what it was, religious standards like "Amazing Grace," "The Lord's Prayer," even jazz or rock. After all, we were a patient-centered service.

None of us was correct. Since the body entrains to a beat, the music needed to have no steady rhythm that would stimulate Peggy's heart, now in the process of shutting down. In fact, if there was irregular breathing—called Cheyne-Stokes, where a dying patient might allow up to a forty-second lapse between breaths—we were to follow that breathing pattern with our music. Our instructor noted that dying was hard work and our music was offered to assist the patient to follow the path where she was already going. Thus, we ought not to employ recognizable melody or words, since they stimulate the memory and bring a patient back to this world.

Carrying only my harp, I walked closer to Peggy's room. Her crying sounded closer to screaming. I entered the room and saw her arms flailing frantically, reaching, then grabbing the bed sheets, the bed railings, her own face. Her grayish hair was tangled and matted from rolling her head back and forth on her pillow, and her eyes searched the room looking for a place to safely light. She was drowning, grasping for a life raft that wasn't there. I had to rescue her. There was a better way to die.

Many of the usual symptoms of active dying were absent. Peggy's hands were not purplish, her skin was not pale or bluish, and she was certainly awake. However, her breathing was irregular and her loud utterances and arm movements could be interpreted as signs of imminent death, possible attempts at contacting the unseen, often family members who have gone before.

I positioned my harp and silently prayed for help. This time I was the one crying, "Help me." I seated myself by her bed and began to play isolated chords in between her outbursts and her gasps for breath in the hope that she could hear the music, perhaps even be distracted. The staff attempted to explain to her that her arm-waving and screaming used up what little oxygen she had, but she was beyond reasoning. Panic and pain were stealing her oxygen.

I quickly decided to change my single-chord approach; instead I would follow her irregular respirations with arpeggiated chords, notes, one at a time, ascending the strings with her inhale, descending with her exhale, then stopping, complete silence to accompany her pauses between respirations. Air in, pause, air out. No regular beat.

I matched her irregular breathing with these slow arrhythmic broken chords for what seemed like fifteen to twenty minutes, long enough for her to respond to the music, but there was no change. I wasn't sure that

Peggy even heard the harp. At this point I sensed that panic, not pain, was the greater of her demons.

I recalled a nurse from Extended Care showing me a gentle technique she employed to soothe patients like Peggy. And knowing that vibration is the transportation for sound I set my harp down on the floor next to me and reached over the bedrails to Peggy. Her actions were so chaotic, so unpredictable. Catching one wild, flying hand, the one nearer me, I held on loosely. Then I placed my other hand over her heart, praying that this intervention might work. I could feel her heart bird-fluttering under my hand. Her other hand continued its manic arcing. I hadn't expected to see anyone in the active dying state fight death so seismically.

Toning a long *Ohhhhhh*, then *Ahhhhhh*, on a low alto note, I prayed the vibrations from my voice and through my hand on her chest would find a healing place in this desperate woman. *C'mon God, I need you here.*

Using the lower notes and specific vowel sounds was the best way to reach her now. No harsh vowels like "eeeeee" or "aaaaaa," no instrumentation, no high-pitched singing, certainly no words. Avoid too much neurological stimulation, as I learned in class. Activating the brain interfered with the spiritual essence of dying.

I continued. *Uhmmmmmm*, then *Ohhhhhh*, then *Ahhhhhh*, repeating and repeating the sequence over and over, ever so slowly. I felt the room discharge some of its tenseness; the toned vowels were relaxing me. But was Peggy feeling them? Too soon to tell, I thought, so I kept on.

More *Uhmmmmmm, Ohhhhhh, Ahhhhhh*. Each syllable as long as my fully exhaled breath. I was a lap swimmer as well as a singer with highly developed breath control, so my extended exhales and my slightly elevated volume overrode Peggy's erratic vocalizations and breathing. On I went, exhaling elongated notes and mustering spiritual energy at the same time.

Slowly things changed. Peggy's noise and activity levels began to decrease. Her free hand, the one grabbing and reaching, descended and lay by her side. She was unable to express herself with words at this point in her dying process, but her eyes focused on mine for the first time, begging for something more. She was still deathly afraid.

Rather unexpectedly, as if I were reading a musical score, my toned vowel sounds changed to a series of chanted words of reassurance. *I am with you. I am with you. Uhmmmmmm.* I breathed and let a little time pass then started up again.

You are not alone. Not alone. Not alone. Ohhhhhh. Ever so steadily and reverently. The improvisation felt like music from the spheres. I still couldn't account for it. Peggy's eyes lost their wide, anxious look, even closed on and off.

Alleluia. Alleluia. Alleluia. Aaaaaahhhhhh. I breathed, paused momentarily. Peggy was silent and peaceful.

My lower back ached and my shoulders were cramped. I had no idea how long I'd been draped around the bed rails. I heard the wall clock ticking, but I didn't shift my eyes away from Peggy to see what time it was. I resumed the soft chanting. Taking a chance, I lifted my hand off her chest to sit up and stretch. Even that small movement caused her to fidget. She moaned. I didn't dare disturb her hard-won reverie so I hunched over again, placed my hand back over her heart, and continued my music.

Kathleen poked her head in the door and I saw that the hall lights had come on. I looked up and softened my chanting, motioning with my head that I thought things were more under control. Kathleen motioned back with her characteristic thumbs up and left the room.

Eventually Peggy fell asleep, succumbing to her body's wishes for oxygen and rest. I cautiously removed my hands from her, straightened up to stand, saw that she didn't move, and slowly left the room carrying my harp. I chanted my way out the door without her stirring. She had lapsed into a deeper state.

~~

It was dark outside when I collapsed into a chair near the nurses' station and let my forehead fall forward to rest on a nearby desktop. Without asking, Kathleen came up behind me and began massaging my shoulders, neck, and back.

"Wow, the music really did the trick. That was hard work in there. You know, the morphine finally arrived but we didn't want to disturb what you had going. And now she doesn't seem to need it."

"I had my doubts more than once. I've never seen anyone fight like this," I said, still enjoying Kathleen's hands kneading my aching body. "Does she have family she's waiting for?" I asked, knowing that despite active dying, a patient will hold on for a special someone to arrive and say a good-bye in person.

"A niece and a nephew from New York City were here yesterday when Peggy was admitted. But no one expected things to go so quickly so they drove back home last night. They didn't seem to have much of a relationship with their aunt. In fact, they were a bit resentful during intake about having to leave work and drive up to admit her to the House. I called them with the latest. They didn't say when or if they were coming back."

"Interesting. And sad, too. There's a story there," I said. Kathleen patted my shoulder.

We would likely never know that story. We observed both loving and appalling events acted out at Hospice when folks were dying. Long-lost friends and relatives showed up. We wondered sometimes if they were hoping for a last-minute bedside inclusion in the will. Greedy, but true. I hoped this wasn't the case.

"I think I'll pack up and head home," I said, easing my head up and sighing.

"Toni's got some mac and cheese coming out of the oven. You want me to get you a plate?" Kathleen was the epitome of the caring nurse. Perfect for Hospice.

"No thanks, but you could get me one of those huge apples I saw in the dining room. I'll eat it in the car."

Kathleen disappeared up the hall to the kitchen area to fetch me an apple while I slid my harp back into its case. As I walked toward the exit, my instruments strapped over my shoulder and tucked under my arm, I stopped to glance into Peggy's open door. She lay on her back, eyes closed. Her chest was rising and falling in easy rhythm, just as I had left her. What a transformation from the chaos I encountered hours ago. And what a blessing I felt to assist this woman into a state of peace, a place where she could ease into a death where grace and dignity replaced fear and pain.

Kathleen handed me a beautiful, shiny apple as I passed the kitchen and then followed me to the door, holding it open as I pushed through with all my baggage. "Be careful of the ice. It's probably refrozen."

"Thanks. That's all I need is a broken arm. No music then," I responded with a smile. I gingerly crossed the parking lot to my car and saw Kathleen shut the Hospice door against the night air.

~~

On the way home I played a Creedence Clearwater Revival CD full blast on the car stereo, singing my lungs out in between bites of the apple. At last I turned down our gravel lane, my headlights lighting up the winding path to our house. The garage doors were open, the lights on. I drove in, turned off the CD player and sat in the car a moment, resting my head back on the seat. The striking silence was suddenly welcome. Gordon emerged from the kitchen door as he usually did to carry in my instruments.

"It was quite a day," I said, "but I think I want to put it behind me for tonight. I'll tell you tomorrow."

"You look beat. I have some chili ready in the crock pot, but I already ate. I'll sit with you unless you want to be alone." He was good about offering me space.

"No, I'd like you to sit with me while I eat. Catch up on your day, the mail, the news."

I ate while he chatted about the day's work on the tractor he was restoring in our barn, the letter from my mother, a call from our daughter Carrie ... all welcome reminders of my other life. I was already looking forward to sleeping late the next morning and taking a long solo walk on our country road once the ice melted.

Tending myself after working with patients was not optional. I had learned this the hard way. During my early internship days I launched right into activities when I got home from a day of offering therapeutic music; no break, no time to process the day's patients, no rest. I wondered why I felt depleted, depressed, resentful, even sick. Seemingly no-brainer tasks like grocery shopping or doing laundry became burdens. Even things I enjoyed felt like too much trouble. Then I remembered my CMP class instructors stressing how hard our work was and how we needed to care for ourselves afterward: a new idea for me.

In hindsight, I remembered wanting to fall in a heap every day when I came in the door from my job as a secondary-school counselor. Some days I wanted to cry or scream. The stakes were high and the emotions charged, but I didn't attribute my reactions to mental, physical, and spiritual exhaustion from hard work. No one suggested that the job was difficult, and no one suggested ways to cope.

I searched out magazine articles and self-help books where the phrase "take care of yourself" repeated itself. But how do you do that? I thought the fatigue, the sleeplessness, the stomach upsets, the anxiety were just me and part of the territory. When you worked, this is what happened to you, and you just endured. I witnessed my parents race through their lives working, volunteering, keeping crazy schedules doing this and doing that, not resting or showing signs of distress. They were critical of people who could not keep up the pace, called them lazy. Was I one of them? What was wrong with me?

I learned in counseling that this tendency to stay busy, juggle many balls at once, was a coping mechanism for numbing my feelings, erasing troubling thoughts. When pushed to the limit this defense mechanism could lead to serious problems. Learning how to take care of myself, after learning who the heck I was in the first place, saved my life.

As I fell into the same pattern of self-neglect in my new work as a therapeutic musician, I recalled the wise words of the CMP instructors and faithfully vowed to continue yoga and walking. I added periods of meditation to quiet my racing mind; socializing with friends became a necessity, not frivolity. Lunches out with a lot of laughs and good discussions weren't a waste of time, but healthful and necessary restoration. Writing out my experiences and feelings every day, journal style, slowed me down and showed me a way into myself. And lastly, I allowed enough days off between trips to Hospice and Extended Care.

"Chili was great. Thanks, hon. I think I'll clean up and then read to relax." We were comfortable reading together most evenings in the silence of the cozy, pine-paneled Adirondack room facing the lake.

A hot shower and warm pajamas encouraged my eyes to close as I read my book. After several attempts to keep my head up and my eyes open, I finally gave up and went to bed.

Sometimes even with exhaustion, intense music sessions played over and over in my head, keeping me awake with tunes I had sung, what had occurred with patients or what I might have done differently. In Peggy's case, I realized in hindsight that I had pushed MHTP Scope of Practice guidelines by using my hands as well as my voice to minister to this dying woman. My heart told me I had done the right thing, the humane thing, that I had trusted my God-given intuition well. Kathleen had observed what I was doing and had no concerns, so I proceeded. With so much on my mind, I was grateful to fall asleep immediately.

~~

I heard the phone ring and glanced at the clock. It was 8:30 a.m. Gordon answered and then handed the phone to me. *Oh, please don't let it be Hospice. I can't do another Peggy day,* I thought as I sat up to take the receiver.

"Hello," I answered, holding my breath.

I recognized Kathleen's voice. "I just wanted you to know that Peggy died early this morning. My shift ended at 10 p.m. and when I left she was still calm, sleeping, non-responsive."

"Did she need the morphine?"

"No, not at all. The night nurse said she just slipped away."

"Did her family arrive in time?"

"They decided not to come. I talked to them this morning and was relieved to tell them she died in peace," she said. "And I told them that our therapeutic musician gave her the best concert of her life."

~~

Every sickness is a musical problem. The healing, therefore, is a musical resolution...
—"Novalis," pseudonym for George Phillipp Friederich Frieherr von Hardenberg,
early German Romantic poet, author, philosopher

Chapter 16

Pachelbel & Patsy Cline

They looked bewildered. So often the caregivers looked bewildered, lost, defeated. Especially the women. This is not a story about one woman or even one man, but a composite of circumstances. I stood in the midst of them, sometimes bewildered myself.

"I made his favorite meal. Brought it from home. Steak, medium rare, the best cut. Baked potato with real butter and sour cream. And a nice fresh Caesar salad," she said, looking me in the eye for an answer. "But he wouldn't eat a single bite."

"I'm sorry," I said, sensing the rejection she'd just encountered. Women so often say "I love you" through food. And the thousands of meals, served over a small intimate kitchen table or around a festive dining room table on special occasions, sustained deep connections over long marriages, partnerships. And now this same loving gesture of a caregiver, a lover to a seriously ill partner, was being turned away.

"He complained about the food here. Everyone knows hospital food's terrible. He wouldn't eat it. I thought a home-cooked meal would help him get back to eating again," she said, covering her face with both hands, finally breaking down into sobs outside his door. She didn't want him to hear her cry.

I wrapped my arm around her shoulder. "Do you mind if I try to explain what's going on? I'm not an expert but I've seen this happen so many times."

"No," she whimpered, lifting her face, then digging into her pocket for a Kleenex.

"He still loves you very much and he loves your cooking too; but his body, his illness are telling him to slow down, eat different foods, or possibly not eat at all. This is natural."

"But if he'd eat, he'd get strong again and kick this darn disease and come home. He wants to come home." She was immersed in denial even though the doctors told her the truth about her husband's prognosis. She wasn't able to hear it.

Who wants to give up?

"Maybe that'll happen, but right now he's actually unable to digest certain foods." I wanted to add that his "wanting to come home" comment might have been his way of telling her he was ready to die. But I held back. She was in no shape to hear it. One revelation, one suggestion, one piece of harsh reality at a time. Dying was not easy on anyone. Her own plate was full, too.

When my father was dying we tried to force-feed him. Dad never missed a meal, and his reluctance to eat his favorites, spaghetti with meatballs, hamburgers, lasagna, confounded us. Until we understood, we sat with him in the hospital with his plates full of food, meal upon meal, trying to coax him to eat, even bribing him with promises of his favorite dessert, ice cream, as if he were a fussy toddler. He wanted to please us, but his poor digestive system rebelled if he ate against his instincts. An informed Hospice nurse offered us a publication called *Gone from My Sight: The Dying Experience* (also known as "The Hospice Blue Book"), which we read cover to cover. The information about eating and food for people in various stages of illness and dying has stuck with me.

Meat—especially red meat—gravy, spicy sauces, heavy casseroles, raw vegetables, bulky foods, were usually given up first. In their place came mashed potatoes, white toast, pasta, bananas, milk shakes, juices, puddings, Jello, scrambled eggs, maybe a grilled cheese sandwich and some brothy soup. Tea took the place of coffee. White-meat chicken or white fish, baked or broiled, might go down well too. And everything in small amounts. Dad resorted to ice cream as his staple food for weeks before he died. And why not?

"Does your husband have favorite foods that might be on the light side?" I asked. "Chicken breast, pasta, mashed potatoes. Think white," I suggested. "But let him decide. And know he might not eat that food either." She nodded, lost in the new information.

I continued. "I can only imagine how it feels, not feeding him or looking after what he eats, especially when he's so sick. But take his lead. That's another way you can show him you love him."

I'm not sure how much she bought the last idea, but I hugged her again and left her in the doorway contemplating my comments. I made a note to get her a copy of *Gone from My Sight*. Perhaps reading the information would help her accept this newest turn in her relationship.

Noticing what was on patients' tray tables, their bedside tables, often led me to the music I chose to play and sing for them. White food, clear liquids, crackers. Eaten food and uneaten food. Each told its own tale about the patient's condition. Light music, like light foods. Maybe a nice easy melody with or without words. Nothing spicy, nothing too exciting.

Oh, Shenandoah, I long to hear you. Far away you lonesome river. Or perhaps *Irene, good night, Irene. Irene, good night.*

Nausea—unrelenting, sickening menace, the body's way of saying "no" to food—and the gradual loss of the ability to swallow usually created the change in diet or the outright refusal to eat. Easing this persistent condition took some doing, some real paying attention. Distraction through familiar tunes with a steady beat, or the opposite tactic, very slow arrhythmic playing or singing, usually eased the malady. A patient's face, the grimacing, the folds around the mouth moving up or down, the wriggling of the body attempting to escape the discomfort, told me which way to go. Another CMP told me he played music with mainly descending notes rather than ascending notes, coaxing, literally pushing down the urge to throw up. I'm now using "Pachelbel's Canon" with its lovely slow descent, its soulful chordal structures moving down toward resolution to ease this malady.

Pretzels, little cookies, soda pop, hard candy, mints, chewing gum—all held clues to the unknowns I so often encountered. Create rest, sleep, ease of breathing, I thought. A steady beat, sometimes familiar. Help patients ignore the nausea or the pulsating pain. Create music with a certain sweetness to help the medicine go down.

Edelweiss, Edelweiss, every morning you greet me. Pure and white, clean and bright, you look happy to meet me.

Clear liquids, tea, ginger ale, hot broth eventually yielded to what appeared to be lollipops, sponges on sticks, moistened with water and swathed into and around a patient's lips and mouth, indicating the most serious conditions or approaching death: patients unable to eat at all, unable to swallow, many times now unresponsive. A bedside caregiver merely kept up the vigil and the comfort level with the sponges as the patient breathed final breaths, mouth wide open seeking dwindling oxygen, eyes closed, body at rest. The sponges led me to pure arrhythmic music, following the irregular respirations of the patient, the music that allowed the natural dying process to proceed gently to its destination. No food, just water. Water music. White music. Nothing colorful.

~~

"It is okay not to eat. A different kind of energy is needed now. A spiritual energy, not a physical one, will sustain from here on." So writes Barbara Karnes in *Gone from My Sight.**

How truly she writes, and how thoroughly I absorbed that lesson.

~~

Back at Hospice, I learned that a new patient's food remained untouched on her tray. Maybe a bite here and there. She was sitting in her wheelchair alone in the Serenity Room when I arrived. Through the glass doors I could see she was skeletal, emaciated. Her name was Sheila. She was only fifty-two years old, not at all near the end stage of her cancer.

The nurses still wanted her to eat.

"She doesn't have much company. I think her refusal of food may be more about depression than cancer. You could try some music with her. I don't know. It's really upsetting all of us to see her starve herself like this," said Kathleen, who didn't force issues with patients. I could hear frustration in her voice. Keeping patients healthy and comfortable was balanced with granting them the right to choose. After all, the residents had few choices left. Sheila chose not to eat.

I opened the Serenity Room door and quietly said hello. "I'm Robin, the house musician." I was taken aback by Sheila's hollow eyes, sunken back into her cheekbones, and her thinning, lifeless, dirty-blonde hair. I waited a few seconds before speaking again.

"This is a beautiful room, isn't it?" There was the brown upright piano

---

* Gone From My Sight, The Dying Experience, by Barbara Karnes, RN. Barbara Karnes Books, Inc. PO Box 822139, Vancouver, WA 98682. Copyright 1986. Revised 2013.

on one wall framed by all the guitars donated in Len's name. The other walls held huge picture windows trimmed in honey-toned oak. One looked out on dense evergreen woods, the other at a sparse rock garden covered with a thin layer of leftover winter ice. It was a sunny day so the room was warm, inviting.

"Do you like music?" I asked, deciding I would get right to the question. Surprisingly, Sheila answered immediately. "Yeah, I like country music. A lot of the old ones. Can you sing that?"

"I sure can, but I might need some help with the words." I went outside the room to fetch my Martin guitar. Its steel strings and gutsy bass would be perfect for country music. I would even use a flat pick. The room was large enough for the bigger sound and Kathleen had indicated Sheila wasn't medically fragile. The space and the patient needed some energy; indeed I had already felt a slight shift in Sheila's demeanor with the mere mention of country music.

I unfolded my chair and sat right next to her and began. *Crazy, I'm crazy for feeling so lonely. I'm crazy. Crazy for feeling so blue.* As I sang the words I wondered why on earth I chose to sing this, of all songs, to Sheila. I almost stopped. But I noticed her lips moving, her eyes brightening.

"That's a favorite," she said. "Mom loved Patsy. Had all her records and played them when she made dinner. I think I know every one. Do you know 'Walkin' After Midnight'?"

"I do." She sang it with me. And then "I Fall to Pieces," "Your Cheatin' Heart." Sheila was right. She knew all the lyrics and the melodies too.

It was funny about playing and singing for depression. I could have gone either way. Play upbeat music to distract away from the blues, or play right into the down feelings with music evoking emotions of sadness. Something led me to choose the latter. It worked. Thank you, Patsy Cline.

Toni, the round, jovial Hospice cook, tapped on the glass doors, then came in to ask if she could make Sheila a sandwich. "I've got your favorite, egg salad. How 'bout it?"

Sheila offered a quick, unexpected response. "Okay. And some chips and a pickle too. What about Robin?"

Toni turned her head toward me. "You want anything?"

I hesitated. "Well, egg salad's my favorite too." It wasn't Hospice policy to feed staff, but Toni must have sensed the urgency for keeping me put for a while longer. The change in Sheila's mood was evident.

After Toni left, we sang more Patsy and then switched over to music from Sheila's era. *It's the right time of the night, the stars are winkin' above.* Then, *Mamas, don't let your babies grow up to be cowboys; don't let 'em pick guitars and drive them ol' trucks.* We laughed about Willie Nelson and Waylon Jennings singing that together.

Then Toni arrived balancing two white paper plates, each holding a bulging egg salad sandwich on white bread along with potato chips and a pickle. I nodded to Toni to put mine to the side as I continued the country music serenade.

Take the ribbon from your hair, shake it loose and let it fall. Layin' soft upon my skin, like the shadows on the wall. Sheila was so wrapped up in the music she might not have known she was taking bites of her egg salad. I didn't dare stop. *Come and lay down by my side, 'til the early mornin' light. All I'm takin' is your time, help me make it through the night.*

I continued playing and singing through her lunch. Her plate was empty when I put my guitar down.

"You didn't eat," she said, rather perplexed.

"I wanted to give you dinner music," I joked. "I'll eat now. How's the egg salad? It looks good."

"I can't believe I ate it all. It was really good. This was like being out in a little café. Music and everything. Thanks."

The egg salad was fabulous and I scarfed it down while Sheila chatted away about other country songs she liked. "How about we save a few tunes for next time," I said, noting that she was looking a bit tired. "I have a big book of country hits at home. I'll bring it."

She agreed and added, "I can't believe I ate my whole lunch. Isn't it funny we both like egg salad?"

We left the room together, she wheeling herself and me walking beside her and carrying my Martin in its case.

"See you next week," I said as she rolled into her room. "Rest up, you've had a big morning." She looked over her shoulder and smiled.

I sauntered up to the nurses' station and made eye contact with Kathleen, who was on the phone. We acknowledged each other and popped a thumbs up sign. I scribbled a note and slid it across her desk.

It read, "You never know what a little country music and an egg salad sandwich can do!"

Chapter 17

Last Words

Saying "I love you"; telling a loved one or a friend how much her life has mattered to you; saying good-bye for the last time; these may be some of the hardest words to utter. For this reason they're often avoided. Ironically, this is when they're most needed. In certain cases, essential. Individuals express these feelings in so many ways besides words: through food, cards, notes, and flowers; visits, calls, gifts, touch, looks. I often say them through music. Dying folks will hang on for that last piece of their life's puzzle to be set in place before they let go.

The Hospice hall was especially quiet that afternoon. Few visitors were present and patients were settled after lunch. Doris and Edgar sat alone in Kurt's old room next to the nurses' station. I poked my head in and asked if they might like some quiet music in the background. Edgar took charge, as I guessed he always had, and responded half-heartedly, "Yeah, I guess that would be okay."

Doris was dying of cancer. They had just celebrated their sixty-fifth wedding anniversary. Edgar was dressed in work clothes, navy blue shirt and matching navy pants. I couldn't decipher the company logo embroidered in red thread above his left pocket, but I saw his name plainly imprinted in blue on a white oval patch on his pocket flap. He wore scuffed black work shoes. Probably steel-toed. I guessed he was in his eighties and that the work clothes didn't mean he was still employed: they were his identity.

Doris, pale and thin, dressed in a faded, loose, cotton-print Hospice nightgown, was lying in bed with the rails up. Surprisingly, her sparse gray hair was freshly set and sprayed. I could see her pink scalp through the tight curls. A volunteer beautician came to the House once a week to cut, shampoo, and style hair, a most generous gift to the bedridden.

A tube ran out from under the bedcovers to a bag attached to the side of her bed. Blood tinged the fluids accumulating in the clear container. The blinds were partially shut, the TV was off. The walls and tables were unadorned with the usual cards, flowers, or photos most patients displayed. Doris and Edgar stared straight ahead in silence.

Everything was bland, beige, flat. The stillness in the room cried out hopelessness, resignation, fear, loss. I felt my energy sag the minute I entered. My hypersensitivity was both my blessing and my curse. I could readily size up a situation only to have its intensity immediately drain me. I had to square my shoulders and inhale a deep, slow restorative breath so that the energy drag passed and I could focus on the task ahead of me. I ascertained that the heavy space in this room was not depression like Sheila's. Patsy Cline couldn't raise the spirits here.

I waited a minute, asking myself what I ought to do.

The staring straight ahead, the dead quiet informed me. I set up my small chair to the side of the room, away from Doris and Edgar, thinking I ought to be as unobtrusive as possible. There was something going on that I was not part of. Cradling the Goya, I began picking a soft gentle arpeggio introduction and played the simple notes up and down the strings without singing, prolonging the lead-in a little longer than usual: I needed to ease in.

I made no eye contact. Then I added my voice. *Let me call you sweetheart, I'm in love with you.* I felt my eyes tear up and a lump rise in my throat.

I wondered if I could continue. But I did.

Let me hear you whisper that you love me too. Keep the lovelight glowing in your eyes so true. I thought I saw movement near Doris's bed. *Let me call you sweetheart, I'm in love with you.* Edgar's hand was sliding across the bedside table, through the bed railing, across the sheet. He grasped his dying wife's fingers. Their eyes remained fixed ahead, and they said nothing. I continued humming the melody softly and slowly to sustain this moment between them.

How could they say "I love you" to each other? The loss was too overwhelming, too emotionally charged, too imminent. It was too risky to break through the silence, the tension. I surmised Edgar was always strong for Doris, held his feelings in check. That's the way he conducted himself. And Doris was strong for Edgar, especially now. How could he live without her? Day after day, sitting around waiting for the inevitable, time moving so slowly, only emphasized the pain. *Let me call you sweetheart, I'm in love with you.* I sang that last line again and ended there, allowing silence to seep into the open space.

The energy changed. Without having to say it out loud, without having to make a big deal out of it, the music allowed Doris and Edgar to say "I love you." No fanfare, no roses, no weighty emotional display, but a simple gesture of touch summarized a deep, unspoken love between them. I hoped that Doris heard those last words through Edgar's touch.

End of life begs for the unspoken to be spoken, for love to be expressed, for gratitude to be offered and grudges to be resolved. This time, as so often, the music had done its work. I was a conduit for the music, the music a conduit for their unspoken feelings. I was blessed to be a witness in the background to a most private, sacred gesture.

When I left, Doris and Edgar were still staring straight ahead without speaking.

And holding hands.

~~

Back at Extended Care, Mrs. Hayden was actively dying. But she was fighting it, the nurses informed me. I immediately went to her room. Her exhausted, elderly husband sat in a chair beside her bed. His wrinkled brown pants and plaid cotton shirt, encased with wide striped suspenders, were nearly threadbare. Mrs. Hayden twisted in her bedcovers in the hospital bed nearby. Her arms flailed and her chest heaved as she called out for who knew what or whom. I figured the Haydens were both in their eighties. Mr. Hayden told me he hadn't slept in three nights expecting his wife to die at any moment. The Extended Care nurses told him she was ready to go.

I began playing the Native American flute to calm her, following her erratic breathing as my studies taught me, stopping my playing along with her long silences in between breaths. This process worked for a few minutes; she'd rest, lay her arms at her sides, close her eyes and seem to let go. Then she'd startle to life, restless arms flying, calling out again, wild eyes looking for something or someone.

She didn't look at me even though I was standing right above her bed.

She was so ready to die; her body had all the signs: mottled feet and hands, irregular breathing, rattling in her chest, no food or water taken for over a week, no bladder or bowel output. She wasn't speaking or communicating in any rational way. But she wouldn't let go.

I switched my music tactic to chanting and humming, took her hand with my hand and placed my other hand over her heart—the magic that had worked so well with Peggy. No luck. A half hour or more passed and I finally got the sense that Mrs. Hayden was willing herself to stay alive. Despite her weakened physical condition her emotional strength was palpable.

I looked over at her husband to see if he might have a clue, but he had fallen fast asleep to the soothing music. At least I did some good, I thought. Caregivers needed music too. The old guy was ashen with fatigue. When I stopped the music he woke up, looking around to find his bearings. I seized the opportunity to ask the question on my mind.

"Could your wife be waiting for someone?"

"Our son might come from New Jersey but he isn't sure. He can't take time off work during the week and it's a seven-hour drive here. He's got a busy family," he said.

It was Friday, the weekend was at hand, I hoped the son would have time off. I decided to offer my two cents' worth. "I hope you'll encourage him to come. I'm almost sure she's waiting for someone to say good-bye. Is he your only child?"

"Yes, and they're really close. He's beside himself to lose his mother."

"Can you tell him she needs him?" I was getting pushy, but this woman was in terrible shape and her poor husband was worn out.

It wasn't uncommon for sons, more than daughters, to stay away when a parent was dying. Facing and seeing the reality can be too difficult. Men are typically raised to stay strong, to hide their emotions.

"I'm glad you got a little nap," I told him before I packed up and went to my next patient. Before I left I reiterated my concerns to him. There wasn't much else I could do for Mrs. Hayden.

Over the weekend I wondered if Mrs. Hayden's son ever showed up and if she passed away. I made a point of finishing writing my patient notes at home so I could drop them off on Sunday and look in on her.

A nursing assistant I didn't know was at the nurses' desk. She was probably a weekend substitute, so I almost didn't ask about Mrs. Hayden. But I decided to inquire anyway.

"Did Mrs. Hayden's son get here?"

"He came in around seven this morning. He drove all night."

"How is Mrs. Hayden doing?"

"Oh, she died about an hour after he arrived," she said matter-of-factly. She most likely had encountered this common occurrence more than once before.

I walked around to Mrs. Hayden's room. The bed was empty, stripped down to the plastic-covered mattress, and the cleaning crew was already preparing the space for the next patient. I stood there thinking about how I had played the wrong music for poor Mrs. Hayden. She was trying to stay alive to hear her son say good-bye, and I was playing music appropriate for dying. She would have been better off if I had played a jig. I was glad she was a fighter.

On a later visit to Extended Care, a nurse took me aside. "You know, after you left, Mr. Hayden went home and got his fiddle. His house is just around the corner. He worried about leaving, but I promised to stay with his wife until he got back."

"Did he play it?" I asked.

"Oh, yeah. He said he liked the music you played, so he wanted to play some music for his wife himself."

"Did you see any reaction from her?" I asked.

"No. When I was in the room and he was playing, she was about the same. Agitated, fighting. Like you saw her. We kept the door closed since that fiddle was loud and he wasn't the greatest player. But he was happy."

"That's great. I think the old guy's music kept his wife alive so their son could get there and say good-bye in person."

"Maybe so. She sure died fast after he arrived."

We turned our heads and caught each others' eyes, simultaneously raising our eyebrows. There was no science to back up our observations. For us there didn't need to be. Our experience was our evidence. We parted in silence.

I strolled down the hall to a solitary patient slumped in his wheelchair. He wasn't dying and didn't appear to be in any pain. Perhaps lonely. But I couldn't prove that. My confidence was a little shaky after misreading Mrs. Hayden.

As I set up my chair beside him, I wondered what I ought to play. Did he want to rest or to be livened up? I asked him, but he only raised his head, still staring at the floor. I took my chances and launched into "Turkey in the Straw," a rousing jig, on my Appalachian dulcimer.

The jig perked him up, he looked at me, grinned and tapped his gnarly fingers on his thigh.

~~

Patients need to say last words, too. My Aunt Marg, who lived in San Diego, suffered a massive stroke that left her paralyzed and unable to talk, swallow, or move her left side. As the matriarch of our extended family, she and I enjoyed a long relationship despite living on opposite coasts of the United States. Our telephone conversations as well as our letters and cards kept us in touch for sixty-six years.

Knowing she was nearing the end of her life, I felt compelled to sing to her. She had followed my musical journey all these years, played CDs from my Mill Run Dulcimer Band days, attended many of my performances, and sang next to me in the church choir alto section whenever she visited. We shared a love of old hymns and gospels.

Her daughter, my cousin Sandy, sat faithfully by her mother's side in the hospital in San Diego. Before I called Sandy, I laid *The American Country Hymn Book* and the blue Presbyterian *Hymnal* by my side. I sometimes needed the words to some favorites, but in truth I figured one song would be enough for Marg, given the shape she was in.

"Sandy, how's it going?" I waited for an update on Marg, then added,

"I'd like to sing to your mom. What do you think?"

I heard her say, "Momma, Robin's on the phone and wants to sing to you. Give my hand a squeeze if you want Robin to sing over the phone to you." There was a new lilt in her voice.

A moment passed. What if Aunt Marg's too far gone for music? What if it's too much for her? How will I know?

Sandy came back, "She gave me a squeeze. I'll put the speaker phone on so she can hear you."

"Sandy, watch for signs of distress, like restlessness, wrinkling brow, a frown, labored breathing. You have to be my eyes. I don't want to make her worse."

I felt awkward singing into a telephone, but I began. *Soft as the voice of an angel, breathing a lesson unheard; hope with a gentle persuasion, whispers her comforting word.* This old gospel tune "Whispering Hope" so often came to my lips when I felt sadness, loss. My aunt was dying. I had to tell her I loved her, and how much I felt loved by her all my life. I hoped she would hear that in my singing.

When I began the next phrase I couldn't believe my ears. In the background I heard strained, mushy attempts at notes and words. It was Aunt Marg singing with me. *Wait 'til the darkness is over, wait 'til the tempest is done; hope for the sunshine tomorrow, after the shower is gone.* I started the familiar chorus, the call and answer line. *Whispering hope, whispering hope, oh how welcome thy voice.* And her frail, musical, nonverbal answer, *Making my heart in its sorrow rejoice,* sent chills up my spine. I was singing for her and for me, lifting both our spirits.

We finished the first verse and chorus and I figured that would be enough. My cousin indicated otherwise. "She's got her thumb up for more." So I sang the other two verses, glad I had opened the country hymnbook to the words. My aunt joined me on the chorus with the alto answer line both times.

At the end of "Whispering Hope" I heard more attempts at singing coming from her over the phone. It was difficult to discern, but Sandy and I both exclaimed at the same time, "I'll Fly Away." I launched into the words and sang all the verses and choruses. Aunt Marg once again tried to sing. But this time she sang harmony with her tired, scratchy voice. I was stunned by her memory and her determination, present in her dying just as they were in her living. I knew she held no doubts about the promises of her religion. *When I die, hallelujah by and by, I'll fly away.* She would fly away to heaven when she died, as the lyrics so aptly proclaimed.

For a full forty minutes, she kept up her feeble harmonization to hymn after hymn. Every time I asked if she wanted more music, my cousin would tell me that her mother gave thumbs up. Curiously, in between songs, while I chose the next number, she went back to her weak version of the chorus to "I'll Fly Away." I knew she liked that song a lot and had heard my band's recorded version a hundred times. Maybe she was honoring our connection this way.

Finally, Sandy thought we ought to end the session. "Momma, you're looking a little tired. Let's stop for now."

"We'll do this again, Aunt Marg," I announced through the phone. "I'll call you soon. I love you."

I heard something in the background but couldn't interpret it. "I think she just tried to say she loves you back," Sandy said.

Sandy cut off the speaker and we chatted, amazed at what had transpired. "She hasn't been this alert since the stroke. She loved it. Did you hear the harmony?"

"Yeah. She's one amazing person. Do you know she never missed sending me a birthday card all these years? Even with your big family and all her involvement with teaching and church and travel. She never forgot me." I choked up.

Sandy heard me break. "We're going to miss her."

We said our good-byes and hung up. The melody of "I'll Fly Away" kept ringing through my head all that afternoon and into the night. I called my Aunt Nan in Boston to tell her the story of her sister. She wept. As I told her about "I'll Fly Away" something clicked.

"Aunt Nan, I know what it means. Marg can't talk, but she's telling us through the melody that we don't need to worry about her. She knows she's dying and she's okay with it. Think about it. 'When I die, hallelujah by and by, I'll fly away.' That's the line she kept singing." I was suddenly moved about Marg sending us comfort from her deathbed with these last words.

"Oh, my God, I think you're right," Nan said.

I ended up calling Aunt Marg two more times to sing. It didn't matter that the words were absent. I sang them for her. Sandy became my eyes each time, watching for any signs that we ought to stop. At the second session all my cousins were present in their mother's hospital room and saw the incredible response she had to the old church music. At times I heard them quietly singing in the background.

The final singing session took place in Aunt Marg's own living room, where she was transferred as per her own written directives, under Hospice care. It lasted only twelve minutes. Sandy held the phone to her mother's ear as I sang her favorites and ended with "I'll Fly Away." There were no more hand squeezes or thumbs up. There was no strained harmony.

"She seems restless," Sandy reported.

"Then I think I need to stop. At this point the familiar music and words can actually call her back to this life. It may be too stimulating. She's transitioning. Can I tell her I love her once more?"

"I'll put the phone back up to her ear."

"Aunt Marg, I love you." I took a deep breath. "Have a great trip to heaven." That last statement seemed to tumble out of my mouth, but as I heard my own words, I felt relief that she was approaching her final reward, as the old hymns call it.

She was flying away.

~~

Observing the delivery of last words from folks involved in the end of life, whether they are the dying patient or the onlooker, convinced me that no matter the means of expressing these testaments, they remain a high priority on the list of how to die well.

My father expressed his love thorough his huge, brown eyes the night he died. He was unable to talk, but his eyes said "I love you" a thousand times over as each of the family lingered one at a time by his Hospice bed in the Adirondack Room for a private time saying our last words.

"Thank you." "I love you." "Don't worry, we'll look after Mom." "You've been a faithful dad and provider." "I'll miss you." And the hardest of all, "I forgive you." Or, "Will you forgive me?" Making amends, putting aside the old stuff, overcoming the fear of seeing a loved one in this state. This is about courage and doing the right thing. There are no second chances for the living or the dying.

Dad waited for calls from family members who couldn't be there in person. He needed to hear them one more time. We held the phone receiver to his ear as they spoke their last words to him. "Grampa, hey, this is Jake. I love you. We had a lot of fun." Dad couldn't answer back but he absorbed their voices. We saw tears form in his eyes as he listened.

He waited for my brother to make a mad dash home from Germany. We all hoped Dad could hang on until Mark walked in the door. "Dad, Mark's landing in Newark. It's one o'clock in the afternoon." Then later, "Dad, Mark's on the train now. He ought to be here in an hour." Whether

Dad comprehended these urgent updates or not, Mark did get his wish to see our father alive, to speak to him, to spend personal time with him.

Not surprisingly, Dad died a few hours after Mark arrived.

There's no documented evidence that these last gestures either by the living or the dying have any bearing on anyone's quality of death or life, but I need no proof. I see the benefits occur over and over.

I know my own life is better for the final moments I spent with my father.

And the last words I said to him.

Whispering Hope

Septimus Winner, 1868

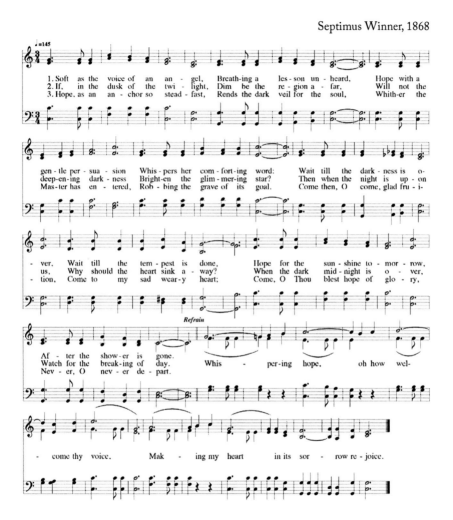

How do we find meaning amidst what appears to be a ruthless and meaningless process? Is it possible to find something redeeming while living with a heartbreaking illness?

—Olivia Hoblitzelle

Ten Thousand Joys & Ten Thousand Sorrows:
A Couple's Journey Through Alzheimers

Chapter 18

Lost

"I can't find my coat. Somebody took my coat. My coat's gone." She grabbed at my arm to stop me in the hallway.

"Have you seen my coat? Can you help me?"

Her mournful crying as she wheeled herself up and down the corridor of her wing in Extended Care visibly agitated the nursing staff and most likely disturbed other patients. It broke my heart. She was lost.

I stopped, resting my hand on her shoulder. "Yes, I can help you," I answered in a direct voice, then asked, "What color is your coat?" thinking she might quiet down and concentrate on the question.

"My coat is gray. I've lost my gray coat. I'm going home today. Can you help me?"

I leaned over her and pulled my harmonica out of my pocket. At that moment a nurse strode by shaking her head, clearly exasperated by Lena's persistent commotion. "I'll see what I can do," I said looking up at the nurse. She shrugged her shoulders and continued walking down the hall.

I hunched over Lena and played a zippy, upbeat folksong directly into her ear, hoping she would recognize it, that it would calm her, distract her from her lost coat obsession.

She turned her head and stared right into my eyes, searching for something. Then she attempted to sing the melody I was playing. Soon her rough, unused singing voice found the notes and she sang along with the harmonica, forming a word here and there. I took the harmonica away from my lips and began helping her sing the lyrics.

Oh, I went down south for to see my gal, singin' Polly Wolly Doodle all the day.

I slowed the pace a bit to help her stay with me. *My Sal she is a good ole gal, singin' Polly Wolly Doodle all the day.*

Lena's face lost its frown, her eyes lit up. She was in the music.

Fare thee well, fare thee well, fare thee well my fairy faye. Could she keep up with the total nonsensical last line of the song? I slowed the tempo way down to give her a chance. *For I'm goin' to Lousianna for to see my Susianna singin' Polly Wolly Doodle all the day.*

She stayed with me on the last line and burst out with a smile, a giggle. Then, she sat up straight in the wheelchair, all full of herself.

"I know that," she said with confidence.

Not wanting her to lapse back into the lost-coat harangue, I launched into "Oh, Susannah," then on to "Way Down Upon the Swanee River" and "Down in the Valley," alternating my voice with playing the harmonica. She knew them all and sang bits of lyrics along with her spot-on melody with every tune I played. We followed the same format. I would play the whole tune through, then stop and sing the song a cappella, allowing her lost memory to retrieve as much as possible. We went on like this for maybe ten or fifteen minutes.

Lena was delighted. And so proud.

The doubtful nurse passed us again in the hallway making our music. There was a new bounce in her step and I heard her faintly humming "Oh,

Susannah." We smiled at each other and heaved a sigh of relief.

I stood up and slid my harmonica into my pocket. Lena began wheeling herself forward as if nothing had occurred between us, but instead of crying out she sang softly to herself. The music had changed her mindset, at least for now.

On another visit, I caught Lena pulling all her clothes out of her dresser drawers and throwing them on the floor. "I'm going home and I have to take all my clothes," she said in all seriousness.

"Oh, I came to sing with you." I began playing Lena's music, the same sequence of songs on the harmonica, then the same a cappella vocals. She looked up, stopped the frantic grabbing and tossing of her clothes and started singing.

I couldn't be Lena's constant musical companion, but the nurses told me that the live music calmed Lena often for hours on end.

"Why don't you just stay here all the time with her?" they asked playfully.

One afternoon when I left Lena's room, a tiny bent-over woman pushing a gray walker with orange tennis balls on the front legs stopped me. "Thank you for coming here. The hallway is quiet and I don't have to keep my door closed when you're here. It's really a shame what happens to people, but they can really be a bother."

"Thank you. You know the music is for anyone. I'd love to come to your room if you ever want your own personal music."

"No, no," she replied quickly. "I can hear it just fine when you're playing in her room." And off she shuffled down the hallway.

I stood thinking about this woman's clear message about her wellness, her mental state. No music for her.

~~

A few wheelchairs were often parked and locked in place along the wall near the nurses' station. The four or five patients in this lineup at

Extended Care were always men. But today there was a woman.

I leaned across the counter of the nurses' station hoping to draw the attention of one of the staff. Phones rang one after the other, call bells buzzed, and the nurses ran in and out of the station to assemble meds, snacks, sodas, coffee to deliver to patients. At last a head looked up at me. I asked, "Who's the new woman out here in the hallway?"

"Oh, Eleanor. She's not new. She's just not talking or eating so we brought her out here with us. Thought this might stimulate her, but there's been no change. We talk to her, offer favorite snacks. Nothing. She's Alzheimer's."

Hearing that phrase made me cringe. Patients were not diseases. They were precious human beings.

"I'd love to sing to her."

"Great," she said lowering her head back to her desk work.

I unfolded my portable chair, unpacked the Goya and seated myself nearly knee to knee with Eleanor. *In the good old summertime, in the good old summertime, strolling down the avenue with your baby fine. He'll hold your hand and you'll hold his and that's a very good sign.*

Her head began rising and I saw the most beautiful, clairvoyant blue eyes find me.

You'll be his tootsie wootsie in the good old summertime.

The words "tootsie wootsie" made her smile, reaching inside that locked brain arousing some deep memory. Was it a lover, the song itself, a summer day? It was summer, but did she know it?

Daisy, Daisy, give me your answer true; I'm half-crazy all for the love of you. She continued to watch me, smiling. And then her lips began moving, fishing around for the words to join me. I slowed the tempo to give her time to capture the most well-known lines of the song. *But you'll look sweet.* I paused again. *Upon the.* I left this part blank to see if she could fill in the word. "Seat" she said, sitting up with authority, delighted with her participation. *Of a bicycle built for two.* We both sang the last line.

After three or so additional songs from Eleanor's heyday, she emerged even more from her hidden place and spoke. "My dad said I couldn't sing. But I sang in the bathroom with the door shut." Her eyes danced.

"You can sing. I just heard you. Do you like baseball?"

She nodded.

Take me out to the ball game, take me out with the crowd. She filled in the lyrics as best as she could, then nearly shouted out *one, two, three strikes you're out at the old ball game,* raising her fingers to count out the numbers. Without hesitation she started telling me more of her story. Her husband was dead, they had no children, but her sister lived nearby but never came to visit.

I felt a tap on my shoulder. Behind me stood several nurses whose eyes were red from weeping. "We never thought we'd see our Eleanor again. And she's back. And by the way, her sister and family come around dinnertime every night."

I left Eleanor chattering away with the nurses. After tending to other patients I made a pass by the nurses' station out of curiosity, eager to see what Eleanor was up to. She still held her head up high and was talking in between receiving spoonfuls of chocolate ice cream from a Dixie Cup, her favorite afternoon snack. She remained alert and talkative for nearly two hours after the musical wake-up call.

Over two years of giving her music, she never failed to recognize me.

"Oh, it's you. Do you have the guitar or the harp today?" she'd chirp as I walked by.

And knowing her family would arrive late in the afternoon, I timed my music for Eleanor so they could glimpse the remembered sister, aunt, cousin or friend who was buried deeply in the recesses of a ruthless, advancing illness.

~~

Eleanor and her relatives were not the only people who were "brought back" by music. An elderly neighbor sent this thank-you note after I had played and sung to him and his wife. He lost his wife shortly thereafter, and he passed away not even a year after her death: a common occurrence.

January 2012

Dearest Robin,

The songs you sing so sweetly, better still using words I can understand and tunes I can recall, even hum to, brought back images of my youthful days when I began chasing girls and forgetting my homework. It's my mind that floods with memories of my momma's soothing voice singing to me in my youth when I was having difficulty settling down or dealing with life's traumas...

Thank you very much,
Kemp Roll

~~

I happened to catch Linda Rains in the recreation office one noontime and asked her about any particular needs of patients. It was rare that we saw each other in that location. She hustled along the four long corridors of Extended Care all day long, disappearing into room after room seeing patients, stopping to say hello, rub their backs, hear their news, look at their photos, distribute mail or magazines. I was touched by her genuine love for her charges, how she remembered their names, their stories. When we were alone in the recreation office together she usually donned a wry smile, then told me a joke she'd heard. Then she'd look at me to make sure I "got" it. I wondered why she felt so at ease with me. I think her jokes kept her sane in that crazy, chaotic workplace. Maybe a good laugh held back her tears when so much of her job involved loss and grief. Maybe she knew I needed a good laugh, too.

"Dave," she said right off the top of her head. "Room 26S. He likes music."

Dave was usually napping when I walked by, but today he was awake. Linda mentioned that his responses could be unpredictable. I didn't ask her what that meant.

Right away I noticed he wasn't very old. Maybe early fifties, even late forties. There was no wheelchair or walker in his room. My heart sank. I guessed he was paralyzed, possibly a paraplegic. So young. Maybe a neurological disorder, or an accident. I shifted my attention away from his diagnosis. Frankly, I didn't need to know details. I was offering music to a human being, not a disease or disability.

Today he appeared to be fairly alert, but he was obviously heavily drugged. His eyes, cast up at the ceiling, were glassy, and a white foamy saliva dribbled from the corners of his mouth. He was stretched out on his bed near the window, clad only in a white undershirt and an adult diaper. His sheets were so askew that only his legs from the knees down were covered.

I introduced myself and asked if he would like to hear some singing and playing. Then added, "I hear you like music."

When he turned his head and tried to speak, his words were slurred and labored. There was no way to decipher them. He sounded like he had food in his mouth. I knew tranquilizers and antidepressants could cause what the staff called "cotton mouth." Many patients chewed gum or sucked on hard candy for it. Dave did neither. A choking hazard for him? I understood the need for an antidepressant, but I wondered why he was tranquillized.

His dark eyes lowered and scanned me head to foot. I felt like they were drilling holes in me. He seemed peaceful and relaxed so I fathomed he would probably fall asleep. That would be fine with me. Those eyes made me uncomfortable. "If you go to sleep, that's okay. I won't be offended. This isn't a concert. Just enjoy the live music in your own room." His eyes didn't move from me.

The staff told me they kept his window curtains open so he could follow the activities on the birdfeeder outside his window. There wasn't much else he could do. I learned that a male staff member installed the birdfeeder for him and kept it full of seed year round. Staff didn't usually put up or refill birdfeeders for Extended Care patients, but Dave was an exception. An empty or filled birdfeeder outside windows gave me clues about which patients enjoyed regular visits from family or friends. Dave's birdfeeder, brimming with seed and eager diners, kept him company, gave him pleasure whether he acknowledged it or not. But I learned he had no visitors.

I slid my chair up next to his bed, cradled my guitar and began to sing. *Sleep my child and peace attend thee all through the night. Guardian angels God will send thee, all through the night.* This was such soothing, low metered music, good for sleeping. But Dave's arms became restless. I had never seen a patient react like that to this song. *Soft and drowsy hours are creeping.* Those dark eyes stared holes in me. He yanked his T-shirt up and scratched his bare, hairy belly.

I continued. *Hill and dale in slumber sleeping.* His hands moved down to his thighs. *I thy guardian watch are keeping, all through the night.*

And then it happened. He thrust one hand down inside his diaper and began furiously stroking his private parts, all the while looking at me. I panicked. Oh, lord. He's masturbating. This behavior wasn't covered in my MHTP classes, and Linda didn't tell me this was one of Dave's "unpredictable" responses. I was undone, unsure what to do. My shock went to disgust, then to feeling sorry for him. He was so out of it he had no idea what he was doing. He would be horrified if he knew. Or maybe he wouldn't.

I chose to look away and keep the music going.

My concentration wandered. A surprising thought occurred. Even patients as disabled as Dave still had sexual urges. What a cruel joke that was. Then I worried that my music had stimulated him, prompted his reaction. Why should I worry about that? Hopefully this man derived some pleasure from life.

Thoughts ran through my head. None of my repertoire was sexually explicit or ever would be. Dave was aroused, that was all.

His primal activity in front of me became more disturbing, despite an inner discussion with myself about this poor deprived man and my surety that he didn't know what he was doing. I needed to leave. Even if he wasn't embarrassed, I was. So I stopped the music, stood up, and left him.

Linda was walking down the hall as I emerged from Dave's room. She must have seen the peculiar look on my face.

"What's wrong?" she asked.

"I was just in playing and singing music for Dave. He began masturbating."

"Oh, is this the first patient you've seen do that? Yeah, they do it all the time. The women, too," she announced matter-of-factly.

"What should I do?" I asked.

"What did you do?"

"At first I just looked away and continued the music. Then I needed to leave."

"There's your answer. Do what you just did. If you can't take it, leave the room."

This time she looked at me with a motherly grin, then continued down the hall.

I had just received another initiation into life at Extended Care.

Did the music do him any good? Would I go back to Dave's room and try again? Was his behavior so common that it didn't faze Linda or other staff? I wondered if I ought to report this to MHTP so patients' sexuality might be discussed in classes.

I was now an advisor to other CMP students and tried my best to prepare them for internship without scaring them or offending them. I would gently report my experience with Dave to them. When MHTP held biannual conferences I networked with other CMPs sharing information, techniques, and experiences, but the topic of patients' sexuality had never entered our conversations. I would bring it up at the next opportunity.

My own feelings told me to ignore patients' reactions, allow them to derive pleasure, healing from my music in any way they could even if it involved sexual responses. I would look the other way or leave their rooms if their behaviors interfered with my delivery of music.

I did go back to Dave's room. Sometimes his eyes, unmoving, staring into me, made me uncomfortable. Mostly he just watched me through a haze from his medications, and fell asleep. He never acted out his sexual urges in front of me again, but I was prepared if he did.

One day a sweet older woman holding a baby doll in her arms, singing and rocking back and forth in her bed as I gave her music, reached below her bed covers to her private places. I continued my music and looked away.

And singin' fee, fie, fiddly aye oh, fee fie fiddly aye oh, oh, oh, oh, fee fie fiddley aye oh ... strummin' on the old banjo.

Perhaps, like staff, I had acclimated to this behavior and accepted it as part of a therapeutic musician's experience.

Chapter 19

The Guessing Game

"We do not recommend playing religious music for patients."

What? These words from our instructor in an early MHTP class stung my ears, didn't make sense.

"We often don't know the patient's religious affiliation, and our organization is careful not to push one religion over another through music choice. Only if the patient requests religious music do we offer it." There was silence in the classroom. Other students must have been processing this new bit of information along with me. So many of our patients were unable to request music.

I thought of my father's love of old hymns and gospels that I sang to him as he eased into his death. He was too ill to select this music, but I saw the comfort, the delight the hymns gave him. In his case, though, I knew his religious preference, but technically he was unable to ask for this music.

With the instructor's words hundreds of songs were dismissed from my repertoire. Worse, the vision of my role at my patients' bedsides changed. I could not imagine pain, illness, dying, loss, fear without the presence of hymns and gospels. I saw CMP work as more ministry than job, but that view was overturned with this information.

I was angry.

Was this a warning or merely a suggestion? An edict or policy? I knew immediately I would work around whatever the pronouncement intended, while respecting MHTP policy.

No one in class asked questions or entered into discussion. Perhaps the other students were devising their own strategies as well. Or maybe not all CMP students cherished the old hymns as I did.

The next week at Hospice I noticed two middle-aged women standing outside Addie's door at the end of the hall. I hadn't seen them before, despite having played and sung for Addie several times. When I first met Addie I fell in love with her: a demure grandmother's face, her soft gray eyes warm and inviting, dear, sweet, Addie seated in her beige recliner. Multicolored afghans spread across her lap in colors similar to the ones draped over my own grandmother's dwindling body at another care facility. Oranges and reds, pinks and yellows, woven in squares intermingled with black and bordered with an odd shade of green. Not colors of my choosing. Leftover yarns from other projects.

Like the finest hostess, Addie welcomed me, offered me a chair, apologized for not having something to serve me. And from that day on, when I ended a music session with her, she apologized for not having money to pay me for my services, despite repeated explanations that I did not accept fees. I was part of the Hospice team.

She was in her early nineties, I guessed, and when I sang for her, a tiny angled smile crept across miles of wrinkles on her face. "I know that one," she'd say. "But I can't sing."

"Did you ever sing?" I asked.

"I sang in the church choir for a long time. Years ago."

That was all I needed to hear on that first visit with Addie to chart the course of our music together. She would love the forbidden music.

"Do you like old hymns?" I asked.

"Oh, yes. Do you know any?"

"Lots, and I love them." Without further conversation I began.

On a hill far away stood an old rugged cross, the emblem of suffering and shame.

She mouthed the words as I sang, an almost whisper escaping her lips. She looked up and away into the sacred space of her life.

I knew from experience that when the eyes cast an upward gaze, visual memory was being invoked. The patient was looking into the distance, re-seeing scenes imprinted from long ago. Likewise, eyes side to side in the direction of the ears, signaled recalling an auditory memory, searching and finding music, words, sounds recorded in memory. Eyes downward could mean retrieving a tactile memory, how things felt on the skin or face or lips, how the hands fingered, smoothed, caressed. It was my pleasure to see these scenes unfold as music opened and welcomed treasured memories.

There's a little brown church in the wildwood, no lovelier church in the dale. No spot is so dear to my childhood as the little brown church in the vale.

Her eyes quickened. Her delicate fingers tapped the rhythm under the open weave of her afghan.

O come, come, come, come; Come to the church in the wildwood, oh, come to the church in the dale; No spot is so dear to my childhood as the little brown church in the vale.

I heard faint humming and nodded to indicate I heard it. She stopped when she saw I noticed her.

"Oh, I can't sing," she said again.

"You just did," I said. "You know if you drink some nice hot tea before you sing, your voice will relax. Do you like hot tea?"

"Yes." She looked like a woman who took tea rather than coffee.

"I'll get you some. Milk, sugar, lemon?"

"Sugar." I had known that, too.

I made a quick trip to the kitchen and asked Toni to prepare a hot mug of tea with one teaspoon of sugar. A tea cup and saucer would have been more Addie's style, but the cupboards held only mugs. More stable for fumbly, shaky hands, I guessed.

Placing it within reach on her end table next to the lounge chair involved moving some reading material. "Days of Our Lives," the daily meditation of so many Protestants, like the one sitting on my grandmother's side table, fell to the floor along with an oversized pair of outdated plastic, light-blue glasses frames. The rhinestones embedded in the yellowed temple pieces caught my eye. I thought to place the material over to her left on the other end table so Toni could put the mug there, but a well-worn King James Bible with bookmarkers drooping from marked pages and a stack of get-well cards occupied that space.

"Can I make a spot here for your cup?" I asked, always careful to respect patient property. "I can put your things on the floor next to you or on your nightstand."

"Right on the floor is fine. I'm so messy these days," she said in her apologetic voice.

"Be careful. The tea's hot," I said after moving her things. Toni set the hot mug next to Addie.

"Thank you," she said in her ever so polite but timid voice. Toni smiled and left the room.

I resumed. *The church's one foundation, is Jesus Christ her Lord. She is his new creation by water and the word.*

She took a tentative sip of the hot tea. Then she mouthed the words to the hymn. Her eyes looked right into me. I felt loved and I loved her back.

~~

The two mysterious women standing outside Addie's door greeted me. "You must be Robin," said the older one, smiling and extending her hand.

"I am."

"I'm Susan and this is my sister, Diane. Addie is our mother and all she talks about is your music. It's the highlight of her week."

As we shook hands and made eye contact I recognized a younger version of Addie in both daughters. They shared her slight frame, small blue eyes, and demeanor of grace; Diane also had her mother's rosebud mouth.

"Your mother is such a joy," I said. "We have a great time with our mutual love of those old hymns."

They nodded.

"I'm trying to coax out your mother's voice. She's very modest, but last week I heard some soft singing. I may have even heard some harmony."

"Oh, yes. She was quite the singer. And a piano player too, mostly at our church," Susan said, then added, "We're here together this week and then we'll be taking turns coming to see Mom. We're wondering if we could join you when you sing to her?"

"Of course. I'd love it. And she would, too, don't you think?"

They agreed with a smile.

"I borrowed two old red hymnals from my church, and your mom and I are going page by page. Our goal is to make it all the way through. I can bring two more of them when I come."

"Oh, we won't sing," said the shyer, less talkative Diane.

I should have anticipated this. There was Addie's voice, her reticence spoken from her daughter.

"It's easy for me to borrow them, in case you want to follow along," I said, suspecting, like their mother, they might sing despite their initial reluctance.

Later that week our quartet of voices in Addie's sunny, beautifully decorated room heightened everyone's spirits, including mine. Susan and Diane reveled in seeing their mother come alive with music.

~~

So many people think of darkness, gloom, sadness when they picture Hospice. Many avoid it, either as potential patients or as visitors, afraid of seeing death face to face, imagining the melodramatic scenes in film, on the news, or worried about their inability to keep emotions in check. I think many are reminded of their own inevitable death and stay away. Ironically, Hospice patients, having come to grips with their mortality, often exude joy, thanksgiving, love. Visitors often witness this acceptance of imminent death as dying patients absorb every last precious moment, fully present, fully grateful.

Hospice, long noted and highly respected for its meticulous symptom- and pain-management, keeps patients extremely comfortable. As experts on end-of-life concerns, in the process of actual death and dying, the Hospice culture also tends to needs beyond the physical. Social workers, spiritual directors, massage therapists, pet therapists, volunteer readers, sitters, therapeutic musicians, beauticians, gently tend not only to the needs of patients but also to those of their families and friends.

When Dad was dying at the lake house, our family availed itself of Hospice literature, nursing assistance, spiritual direction, and social workers' advice; round-the-clock help was a phone call away. He never suffered once he went under Hospice care. After his death, we attended counseling groups with others who had recently lost a loved one. My mother especially felt the comfort of others in her group who understood the grief, the loneliness of fresh loss.

Children's groups addressed the needs of younger family and friends of the dying, fully informed that various ages held different beliefs about what happens when someone passes away. Age-appropriate discussion and activities dealt with fears and misconceptions rather than accept the notion that "They're only kids," a common dismissal from overwhelmed, grieving adults.

~~

Addie and I didn't make it all the way through the red hymnal. She faded further into her illness and slid into non-responsiveness. I continued to sing her favorite hymns, but slowed the tempo down to match her measured but stable breathing. Her daughters alternated visitation weeks and then, near the end, came together to stand by their mother's side. They sang with me during my last visit to Addie, using the old red hymnals for words. The only request I made of them was to return the borrowed books to the nurses' station when they weren't using them anymore. I hoped that they would sing to Addie even when I wasn't present.

Early the next week when I arrived to do music at Hospice, I saw a stack of three red books placed on top of the nurses' station desk. I stopped for a second and took a deep breath. Moving closer to the station I noticed a white envelope sticking out from under the cover of the top book. I opened it and recognized my name written neatly on the envelope, so I slid it out and opened it. Enclosed was a touching thank-you note signed by both Susan and Diane, and a generous gift card to a local, highly regarded restaurant. I was taken aback. Holding the note and gift card, I walked down to Addie's room looking for her daughters. It was empty, stripped of the wall hangings, the pillows, the colorful afghans. Susan and Diane had already collected their mother's things and left.

I stood outside Addie's room and pondered whether I could accept the gift card. Taking such offerings from patients or family was not in line with Hospice policy, but I was not paid staff. Susan and Diane knew that I essentially volunteered my musical service to their mother. I even wondered if Addie herself had put them up to this last gesture. That would be so like her. I recalled her repeated concern after our music sessions that she had no cash with her to pay me—despite my saying that payment was not part of the deal. As I walked back toward the nurses' station I vacillated between enjoying the gift and sending it back to the donors.

The thought of returning it felt like cruelty. I had come to know Addie's daughters well enough to understand they would be upset by the return of the gift. Rather than spoil their remembrance of our interactions with their mother at Hospice, I decided to keep it.

Realizing that Kathleen might have noticed the white envelope sticking out of the red hymnal, I was not surprised by the knowing look she gave me when she saw it, now open in my hand, and I asked her for Susan and Diane's addresses. We did not exchange words, but merely acknowledged each other with a nod.

"I guess that's the end of that," I said breaking the unusual silence. Right then my struggle over taking the gift card gave way to the reality of my loss. That was the end of it. My hymn-singing buddy was gone and now, for a moment, I was lost. I began to cry.

"This is hard work," I blubbered. Kathleen came around the nurses' station and we hugged each other before she moved down the hall to answer a patient's call button. I tucked the envelope under the cover of the top hymnal and walked over to unpack my instruments. Except for Addie's room, the House was full.

In the afternoon, when I placed the hymnals and the envelope into my satchel, I thought about how the messages of those old hymns assured Addie and her daughters of her heavenly ascent, her reunion with family and friends, in a life ever after that she believed in.

I could take comfort in that.

~~

I continued to develop my own policy about singing religious music.

Luckily my repertoire included a varied selection of music encompassing many faiths. My choices were often the result of a quick scan around patients' rooms for religious icons, a cross with a Christ figure, or an empty cross, Roman Catholic and Protestant; a Star of David, a Bible, Koran; pamphlets, books, rosaries and medals, feathers and dream catchers.

I also came to realize that most of my patients knew "Amazing Grace" or "In the Garden," songs that I believe are planted in both the sacred and the secular traditions. Singing those songs became my test cases as I searched for clues about religious traditions and preferences. They elicited more information from patients than any other music I played: tears of remembrance and of home, of someone singing those very songs to them; stories about their churches, religious experiences. Their responses led me to direct questions to them about music choices.

"Do you like the old hymns, Gospels? Or do you have any religious affiliation?"

I've been asked to sing both versions of "Ave Maria" and "The Lord's Prayer," plus countless other religious music to people who are religious and nonreligious. The melodies and the messages, pop music of its day, go straight to the heart.

I was relieved to find my way into the MHTP policy without compromising either their philosophy or mine about whether, and how, to offer religious music.

~~

A new experience occurred when Hillie's family asked me to come as a private caregiver to her home. Their mother was dying, and they resolutely wanted hymns for her. Mostly non-responsive and stretched out on the living room sofa, Hillie lay wrapped in a comforter and propped on all sides by large bed pillows. Her eyes were open. Glasses of water with bent straws leaning against their sides, brown pill bottles and crumpled tissues cluttered the end table nearest her head. As I unpacked my guitar, her eyes followed me with suspicion.

Despite knowing she wasn't responding verbally, I posed a question. "Hillie, your family has asked me to come today to sing hymns to you. Would you like that?" I waited for any indicators. There were none, but her eyes remained fixed on me. I went on, "I'll sing and play for you, as your family has asked. Very softly, very easily. And I'll be watching for any signs that I ought to stop."

No response, so I raised my guitar and began. *Nearer my God to Thee, nearer to Thee; E'en though it be a cross, that raiseth me.*

She kept her eyes on me and remained expressionless. Her family sat around the living room listening, glancing back and forth between me and their mother, then among themselves. They were pleased and relaxed with the music. I continued into one of my favorites, its lyrics so fitting for this setting. *When peace like a river attended my way, when sorrow like sea billows roll.*

Hillie didn't move, but other heads nodded to the music. Her breathing remained steady, and her eyes eerily stared at me. I felt like I was singing to a corpse. Hillie showed no reactions whatsoever. Was the music completely unreceived? How would I know what was going on with her, what she needed or didn't need? The family members were involved in the music, happy for providing something special by inviting me to give music to their mother. But it wasn't about them. Or was it?

I sang on. *It is well (it is well), with my soul (with my soul), it is well, it is well with my soul.*

I played and sang for about thirty minutes, our agreed-upon time, then decided to end with "In the Garden."

I come to the garden alone, while the dew is still on the roses. Hillie responded by creasing her brow, then with restlessness in her hands and feet. She reached up with one hand and pulled at her throat.

I watched carefully, but went on, *And the voice I hear falling on my ear, the Son of God discloses.* I got the feeling that Hillie was disturbed, agitated with this music so I stopped.

"Oh, keep going, she loved that song," said her daughter. "We love it too."

"I'm seeing signs of distress, I don't want that," I responded and put down my guitar. I wouldn't ask any questions about her history with the music, and there would be no more music. I felt very uncomfortable, fearing the song had gone too far into her memory, her emotions. There were no tears, and I wondered if she was expressing anger with her actions. Her eyes didn't tell any tales even though she still kept her gaze on me.

I knew she was a tough, well-educated woman from a prominent Dutch family from the Amsterdam area of upstate New York. She had been a nurse, and her husband, another stoic Dutchman who had died years ago, the village doctor. Expressing emotions, especially with a stranger, was not part of that equation. The music probably pushed that limit. Her family, seated nearby, didn't exhibit any emotional reactions either.

"Well, that was nice. I'm sure mother enjoyed it. Will you come again?" asked the younger son.

I was conflicted, really didn't want to put Hillie or myself back into another difficult situation. In my heart I felt the music was not her thing, but it certainly was the family's thing.

"Let's see how she does later today. If she sleeps well, shows no distress, I'll come again. Next time I'll stay away from certain music."

I called the family later that evening to check on Hillie. They cheerfully reported she had fallen asleep and shown no signs of pain or upset. We set up the next appointment. I knew I would stay safe: sing popular music from her era in the '30s and '40s, well-known folksongs, maybe just bring my harp and play without any singing at all. Unfamiliar music.

When I arrived, Hillie was in her bedroom lying on her back, nicely tucked in with a pale green comforter bordered with embroidered wild flowers. I knew she was an avid gardener and suspected a family member had carefully chosen this bedcover. Her eyes were sleepy this time, half-closed, and she didn't open them further when I spoke to her. Her sons and daughter stayed out in the living room rather than come in close-by for the music.

"We can hear the music just fine out here," the daughter reported. I wondered if the last session of music had aroused their emotions and made them uncomfortable like their mother.

I hummed tunes to "Bicycle Built for Two" and "Sidewalks of New York," then sang the lyrics to "You Are My Sunshine" and "Over the Rainbow." I kept the tempo down so Hillie would not rouse. Her eyes closed all the way and she slept for the last verses of "Rainbow." To accommodate her sleeping I changed tactics, switching to the harp and plucking out slow Irish melodies, lesser-known ones so she wouldn't stir. She awoke anyway. I saw her wrinkle her brow, saw her hands and feet twitch beneath the quilt. Then one hand pulled out from under the covers and grabbed at her throat.

I took my hands off the harp strings and observed. I was unable to read Hillie's responses.

Again, the family, from the living room, gushed about how the music was so beautiful, so relaxing. "We love that harp," said a son. "Are you going to play more of it? I bet mother is pleased." *Yes, the music is perfect for you*, I thought, *but not for your mother*.

"I'm not sure this is right for her," I said, going on to explain. I realized they hadn't been able to see their mother during the music both times. All they knew is that they enjoyed the music and that they were offering a loving gesture to their mother.

They were paying me, and paying me handsomely. I didn't want to think about money and finally packed up and ended the session. They insisted on a full fee, plus tip. We agreed they would call me if they thought more music was in order.

Thankfully, I didn't have to fake it when they called to ask for a third session: my schedule was booked. But I decided I wouldn't return, as it was clear that I was giving the family members music, not their dying mother. That felt like cheating.

Hillie died easily, without music, a few days after I declined the invitation. To this day whenever we see each other, the family tells me how special the music was for their mother.

I get an uneasy feeling thinking about my music experiences with Hillie. So many unknowns. She remains one of the most mysterious patients I've encountered. I've talked about her with colleagues, hoping for insight. All we can agree on is that our work is often a guessing game.

Maybe staying in the mystery is itself the lesson.

Chapter 20

Chaos and Clarity

My friend Jane talked about Grace.

"She's back in the hospital again," she said over lunch, talking more to others than to me. I was a newcomer to the Friday lunch bunch at the café in the small village of Northville in upstate New York. I knew nothing about Grace, only that her name appeared in the church bulletin on the prayer list week after week. At lunch the next Friday Jane mentioned Grace again.

"The cancer's back. Mike's devastated."

I could see Jane was devastated, too. I finally spoke up. "Can you tell me who Grace is?"

"She's on her third recurrence of cancer. She and Mike live on Bridge Street. Much younger. I think Grace is under fifty," said Jane. "They were a few years behind me in school."

That was my introduction to Grace and Mike and their harrowing dilemma. When I drove by their well-kept white clapboard house on Bridge Street I thought about Grace and the misery she might be going through. I knew it all too well.

~~

My own narrow escape from cancer began at age thirty-nine, when a large hard mass rose up in my right breast. My own fingers found it. Within days of its shocking discovery, my breast and all the lymph nodes in its vicinity were removed during an emergency surgery.

When I found the mass, my husband and I were living in northern Virginia, but "homeless." Our new house was way behind schedule. Our old house had sold quickly so we had to move out, gypsies begging for a place to set up our tents. All summer we camped at my parents' home, sixty miles south near Fredericksburg off Interstate 95, more than an hour from Gordon's work, our doctors, friends, church, and the kids' playmates and schools. Summer was ending and our three kids were entering new schools—one to kindergarten, one to middle school, and the oldest a freshman at a science magnet high school.

Our plan was to extract ourselves from my parents' over Labor Day weekend to be ready for the start of school the following Tuesday. A dear friend offered her finished basement closer to our new home for another campout, a brief stay while we awaited completion of our house. I would provide the kids' transportation to their bus stops since we were still out of our own schools' boundaries.

At the first meeting with the surgeon, on the Friday before Labor Day, I heard him utter shocking words as he described my pathology report: monster, killer, fast-growing, aggressive. And then mastectomy. With the last word, time stopped. I took a deep breath to start it again. Even though his frank descriptions caused me to begin trembling, I gathered myself together and spoke calmly. "Can I have surgery in a week or so? We're moving tomorrow and we need to get the kids into school next week. And my husband starts school too."

I'll never forget how the surgeon slid his arms across his desk, leaned forward and stared me down. "Do you want to live?"

"Yes," I answered timidly, now shaking all over, and turning my head to see Gordon's stunned expression.

"You and your husband report to the hospital tomorrow at 5:30 a.m. I have the O.R. for 7 o'clock. Someone else can move your belongings."

With that he rose, gathered my paperwork, and stepped toward his office door. "See you in the morning. And don't forget to follow pre-op instructions," he said and closed the door behind him. When he left, I grabbed Gordon for dear life. I don't know if he wept, but I'm sure he felt my chest heaving and heard me crying, "No, no, no."

My children acted out their fears as I endured the aftermath of surgery and the ravages of chemotherapy. The kindergartener later expressed in therapy that when my husband coaxed him into the dark bedroom where I lay in a nauseous agony to kiss me goodnight, it felt like a haunted house. It scared him to death, poor baby, and I couldn't help him. My daughter, the middle-schooler, threw herself into her own passions, ballet and school, and stayed away from the house as much as she could. My older son found solace in the church youth group, jazz band, skateboarding and, we later found out, marijuana.

My husband, a reliable, steadfast Midwesterner, dug into running the household, transporting the kids to activities, and going to work even after nights of emptying buckets next to my side of the bed after I heaved and heaved from chemo.

And I, typical of my personality, tried to be strong, upbeat, involved, the wife and mother everyone was used to. I kept silent about my terror of dying, my increasing anxiety, my dread of chemo, and the black depression creeping over me. My insides were crumbling while my outsides smiled and managed to push through.

~~

Grace and her house ignited all these memories.

Mike had married Grace, his high school sweetheart, as soon as they graduated and started his own flooring business. Now he was adrift, battling alcoholism, trying to stay clean for Grace, but he had few resources for his sanity or his sobriety in the little village.

Like us, Grace and Mike had three kids. The youngest, their eighteen-year-old son, was disappearing for days, drinking and drugging heavily with some older guys. He was a senior at the high school and had lived his young life on a bed of coals, watching his mother's life come and go as she battled the cancer over and over. I assumed he was unable to express his emotions, his fears, his grief, so he ran off to escape the reminders at home. The two daughters were married with young children and lived nearby.

During Friday lunches Jane talked only about Grace's outsides—how strong she was, how upbeat. I imagined her insides. When a Hospice nurse called and asked me if I would make a house visit to a new patient on Bridge Street, I was grateful: I rejoiced that I might get to offer healing music to Grace—to her outsides and her insides.

Their blacktop driveway was full of vehicles. A white van and a large black muscle truck with doors painted with Mike's flooring business logo were parked in the back. I assumed the other cars belonged to family and friends. I slipped my Passat wagon into a space just wide enough to open the car doors and retrieve my instruments without dinging anyone's paint job.

They were expecting me, so my knock on their side door, the one Mike had asked me to use, was answered promptly. From the driveway I had seen a red-and-white oxygen sign and a note tacked to the front door. I heard a dog barking incessantly in the background, and as soon as a man opened the door a wall of cigarette smoke hit me in the face and more loud noise escaped the house.

"I'm Mike. You must be Robin. Come on in." He could see my hesitancy as the large, angry-sounding dog came closer to me, now growling in between barks. "He won't hurt. He'll stop barking once he gets to know you."

"Hi, Mike. Thanks for inviting me over," I said, still eyeing the dog.

Mike was a rough-looking man, unshaven with beat-up hands, dressed in blue jeans with threadbare knee and a green flannel shirt with the two top buttons left open to expose a hairy chest. His blondish hair was buzzed short and he held a lit cigarette between his fingers. Thick lenses in his gold aviator glasses magnified his tired, bloodshot eyes. I imagined he had not slept well for days. Maybe weeks.

"Yeah," Mike said. "Grace might like some music. Her bed's in the living room. The girls and the baby are in there with her."

I passed through the kitchen where two women sat smoking and drinking coffee around the kitchen table. Their ashtrays were overflowing with butts. They gave me a passing glance but didn't stop their conversation to greet me.

The source of all the other noise became apparent when I entered the darkened living room. Two younger women were talking above a twangy country singer blasting his music over a fully amplified band on the large television. A toddler chased after a ball she was throwing across the living room, screaming with glee. The husky dog followed me into the room and continued its threatening barking. I heard squawking, near shrieking, and followed my ears to the corner of the room where two large black bird cages dominated the space. Three parrots sat on perches adding their two cents' worth to the cacophony. My nerves were jangled immediately and, pulling myself together, I wondered how I would tackle the situation. Surely Grace would like some peace and quiet.

A tiny, wasting woman lay slightly propped up in a hospital bed jammed against the front entry door. Tubes ran from her nose to the oxygen concentrator whose hissing and popping added staccato beats to the chaos. Her head was bald with small wispy patches of hair trying to grow back after who knows how many rounds of chemo. I thought how, by some luck, I had not lost my hair during my chemo and wondered how many times Grace had lost hers. A catheter tube fell from under her sheets to a bag hitched on the side of the bed railing. I took note that the urine bag was full and the urine was dark yellow, but not blood-tinged or brown yet. Grace had some time.

She looked up. Her skin was gray, shriveled. She was aged beyond her years. I strained to hear her speak over the noise.

"Thanks for coming," she said blinking watery eyes to focus on me. Then she directed her comments to her daughters. "Can you turn off the TV?"

One less layer of noise calmed the scene a little.

I noticed a small open container with a white plastic spoon stuck into what looked like applesauce on the bedside table next to her. Grace was still able to swallow. Amber pill bottles sat next to it, most likely pain meds dispensed by Hospice. Pain management, a forte of the Hospice organization, sought to address a patient's discomfort before it became overwhelming. Meds were offered more liberally than in most hospitals and nursing homes. Oral pain meds, administered with the help of the smooth texture of applesauce or pudding, allowed patients to continue to swallow the longer-acting pain pills. First the pills were taken whole, then crushed as the patient became less able to swallow. The final pain med, oral morphine, was deposited through a small dropper under the tongue or to the inside of the patient's cheek. Two drops every four or so hours, and then every two hours, then as often as needed until the end.

I had participated in this pain-management activity while my father descended into his final stages. Even with congestive heart failure, he never panicked as his breathing capacity diminished with the accumulation of fluid in his lungs. He didn't wince in pain or struggle with breathing as his body shut down, one organ at a time. The morphine, lovingly dripped into his system from my hand or the hands of the round-the-clock nurses we hired, kept him pain-free and comfortable until his last breath. I hoped this would be the case for Grace.

"May I set up my chair here next to your bed?"

She nodded and asked her daughters to lower the hospital bed so she could put her head back to listen.

"I'm not an entertainer and expect nothing from you," I said. "If you fall asleep in the music, it would be just right. I'll keep playing and singing as you rest unless I see signs of distress. If you don't find the music pleasing or if you feel you've had enough, let me know. I'm not offended. This is just for you."

The dog finally stopped barking and went into the kitchen. The daughter with the toddler said good-bye and eased through the crowded space to leave, while the other daughter got up and went into the kitchen. I hoped I had not blocked them in with my car. Mike appeared and stood in the background watching me and Grace as I began playing. He had the air of a protector, a man who had learned to take charge over the years during his wife's recurring illness. He also exuded sadness and fear.

Once the TV was off, the only light in the room came from a small lamp and a glowing cell phone on the bedside table with the pill bottles. Thick drapes covered the windows. I felt trapped in the heavy cigarette air, by the darkness, and by the threat of sudden unpredictable shrieks from the nearby parrots.

I wanted to soothe Grace's nerves, to allow her to rest, but I was certain that wasn't going to happen in all this mess. I began singing. *Love me tender, love me true, all my dreams fulfill.* Grace listened. Mike came around to the chair his daughter had vacated and sat down.

"She likes that song," he said, looking at his wife. Their eyes met. I hoped this song would not be too much for them. For *my darling I love you and I always will.*

I finished "Love Me Tender" and moved on to some gospel and country tunes, slowing the usually lively tempos but keeping a steady 4/4 beat, the rhythm of the heart, of walking, of comfort. Grace closed her eyes, settled into her pillow, and seemed to relax. I felt my shoulders fall and my neck loosen, finally settling in myself. Maybe I could actually bring peace.

Then the cell phone rang and startled us all. Mike answered. The phone roused the parrots, but no one made any effort to hush the birds. After the phone conversation, I noticed Mike replaced the phone in the same place so it could interrupt again at any time. I appeared to be the only one bothered by the noise—or the smoke, which was prompting my nose to run and my forehead to start aching.

I played and sang some familiar hymns, and Grace closed her eyes again. I'm not sure she went to sleep, but she did seem peaceful.

"She's breathin' easier," Mike observed.

"The steady beat of the music can actually do that," I said.

"Really?"

"I'm wondering if you have some CDs you could play for her with that nice, easy, one-two-three-four beat to them. Not too fast. Or loud."

"Yeah, I think we got something like that," he said. I could see him thinking about the CDs already.

"The country music these days is so ramped up it might make her anxiety and her pain levels go up. And it could make her breathe too fast."

"Yeah, she likes country, but maybe not now." He was invested in the new ideas. Progress.

Grace's eyes remained closed during our conversation. The oxygen concentrator clicked more slowly with her easier breathing. I wondered why she didn't choke or cough in the smoke-laden air. The cell phone rang again but she didn't stir. The parrots shrieked and the dog began barking as I stood up to put my guitar in its case and collect my coat. Still Grace slept.

"I'll call you about making another visit if you think this has been good for her," I said.

"Yeah, I think so. What about later this week?" he asked, ever the vigilant husband seeking any interventions that might help his wife. I also sensed the urgency in his request. He knew that this time Grace was dying.

I backed out of the driveway onto Bridge Street and turned home toward the lake house. The atmosphere I had just left disturbed me. I knew I would never want anything like that for myself, and I didn't want it for anyone else either. But Grace had chosen to leave the hospital to come back to this: smoke, dog, parrots, kids, family, television, phone. And it became clear to me that it was not my job to change it or judge it. What I called chaos, she called home.

When my own cancer surgery was over and we finally moved into our beautiful new, bright, quiet house I was terribly lonely and scared. On a Saturday afternoon a pair of gifted teenage musicians from church set up their chairs and music stands in my sunny bedroom where I lay weakened and worn down from chemo. The children's music director had sent them my way. They called themselves The Grand Duo and serenaded me with classical music arranged for flute and classical guitar. It was lovely, uplifting, joyful. I felt cared for, wrapped in sumptuous healing music. That was my kind of soundscape, my kind of atmosphere. Grace had her own preferences and I respected them.

A few days after my first musical visit to Grace's home, I called to arrange a second visit and was readily invited. Mike met me at the door along with the same annoying sounds and smell. But things were different. The TV was off and a CD player next to Grace's bed sent the smooth, slow rhythmic sound of Frank Sinatra's voice into the room. Grace was awake but fully relaxed.

"I did what you said. I found some music for Grace. She's been a lot more settled down." Mike's eyes brightened. He was proud of his success.

"I'm so glad. Maybe the live music today will give her even more pleasure."

I sidled up close to Grace's bedside and played and sang movie tunes: "Somewhere Over the Rainbow," "Raindrops Keep Fallin' On My Head"; I followed them with some John Denver: "Annie's Song," "Sunshine On My Shoulder." Then I hummed the theme from "Love Story" and watched her slowly turn her head and smile at Mike. As I offered this music I took note of other changes in the scene since my last visit. The tube carrying urine from Grace's body to the bag by her bed was tinged brownish red and not very full: her kidneys were shutting down. There were no amber pill bottles or open applesauce containers on the side table: she was now getting liquid pain meds. And she was extremely limp. She did not speak.

Her breathing was steady, so I kept my tempo within the normal 50 – 70 beats-per-minute range, not wanting to speed up or slow her respirations. Like last time, Mike hovered close to keep watch over his precious wife.

I was fully aware that this might be my last chance to offer music to Grace. All the signs of an imminent death were present except the irregular breathing. I sang and played on, adding hymns and slow country, mostly omitting the words to songs and just humming or toning the tune. Other times I made up melodies and played chord sequences on the guitar. Grace slept. At one point I glanced over at Mike, and saw through his thick glasses that he was weeping. He didn't try to hide his face or pretend to be a tough guy. He was visibly broken, shaken, moved to tears. I was relieved he could allow himself to cry in my presence.

I may have stayed for an hour. There's no sense of time in these situations: I'm not on the clock. When I stopped the session, Mike got up and came over and hugged me.

"This has been real good for Grace."

But I knew it had been real good for him, too.

"I'll call you about another music session. And that CD music you chose for Grace is just perfect."

He beamed. When life is so out of control, having one tiny intervention to offer means the world. He could do something for Grace when there was nothing else.

Three days later I received a call from Hospice.

"Grace died in the night. Mike wants your phone number. Can I give it to him?"

"Sure. Thanks for the call. I hope things stayed calm."

"Yes. Mike and the whole family were with her."

I expected Grace to die, but there's always some thread of hope for a miracle, especially when the patient is so young. I had gotten my miracle at age thirty-nine. Grace wasn't so lucky.

Mike called later in the day. "Can you sing for Grace's memorial service?"

"I can. I'm honored. Do you have any music in mind?"

"Maybe 'Amazing Grace' and some of the other church music you sang."

"Do you want some harp music before the service?"

"Sure. That'd be okay." I could hear the exhaustion in his voice.

I didn't have the heart to tell him I charged a fee for memorial services. Jane mentioned at lunch on Friday that Mike had not been taking any flooring jobs for the last few months so he could spend every minute with Grace. So I let the idea of a fee pass.

The service was simple, sweet, short. I played and sang my part as agreed upon. I was happy to see the errant son sitting next to his father and wondered if he was at his mother's bedside for her death. After my last piece of music and as the church emptied, the minister approached me and handed me an envelope.

"What's this?" I asked.

"Someone wanted you to have it."

"Who?"

"They didn't want to be named. Just take it."

I tucked the envelope into my purse, packed up the guitar and harp, and walked out to my car. Settled in the driver's seat I sat a minute, thinking about Grace and the service. So sad. Out of curiosity I reached for my purse and fished out the envelope.

There was cash but no note.

I started the engine to drive home and saw Jane walking from the church to her car. We waved. I almost stopped to roll down my window and speak to her, but she wasn't the kind who wanted thanks or praise or recognition. She just gave from her heart.

So I drove on.

~~

It is our work only to understand our own suffering and, therefore, be available at deeper levels to those we serve.

— Stephen Levine, *Who Dies?*

Chapter 21

Teeth and a Sweatshirt

The first thing I noticed about Ruth was her shoes. Large men's Reeboks, soles propped upright on the footrest of her recliner, like the gas and brake pedals on my car. As I came closer, I saw ballooned ankles encased in white athletic socks, overflowing from the tops of the massive black shoes. Both a walker and a wheelchair were parked to the side of her wall. She sat alone in a private room at Extended Care.

Then I noticed the newspaper fanned across her chest, nearly obscuring her head. Unkempt gray hair, a pinkish, wrinkly forehead, and glasses on a large nose were all that were visible. She lowered the noisy pages of the paper to her lap.

"I read *The New York Times* every day, every page," she announced in a loud voice, looking me in the eyes.

"Oh," I said, not knowing what was coming next.

"Do you read?" she asked.

"Yes, but not the *Times*. We haven't decided on a paper yet."

"Are you going to sing to me?" she asked, looking at my guitar and folding the paper in half, then into quarters, finally laying it across her lap and smoothing it flat.

"You can still read the paper if you want to," I said. "I'm Robin, the Extended Care musician, and I thought you might like some music this afternoon."

"I think I would. Have you been on the other hall to Robert's room?"

"Yes, I sang for him last week."

This time I could see something was coming.

"He's my husband, but he makes me so mad I don't even go over to see him anymore. He won't talk to me. I don't even think he knows me. Just sits there looking at me like I'm nobody."

I knew what she meant. Robert was completely lost in advanced dementia. He was one patient the music couldn't awaken, just sat there, staring ahead. I understood her anger. But it felt more like grief.

"Yes, Robert's pretty quiet. I know what you mean."

"Married sixty-eight years and now he treats me like this."

She was a tough one. Her hands, like her feet, were large. Knuckles like burls on a tree limb. I wondered if those hands had worked in one of the local glove factories, the only outside work women of her generation could find in rural Upstate New York.

"I'm ninety-five," she said. I raised my eyebrows, nodded, and began singing. *Summertime and the living is easy, fish are jumpin' and the cotton is high.*

I jazzed up this great song for her and soon her hands and feet were moving to the music. *Your daddy's rich an' your ma is good-lookin'; so hush little baby, don't you cry.*

I was swaying with the music myself. Ruth and I were smiling at each other, delighted in the moment. I brought the song home and improvised some high slides with my voice, adding more jazz guitar underneath. She loved it. So did I.

"You got a great voice, honey. You know any hymns?"

That's all I needed. "I bet you know this one," I said.

I come to the garden alone. She immediately shed her guard, became still, and looked out in the distance, a sure sign there was a memory passing right in front of her. *While the dew is still on the roses.* But she didn't shed a tear, as so many patients do when they hear this music, these words.

"I'm a Lutheran," she proclaimed before I could even get to the chorus. "I haven't been to church in years. Sometimes I go to the service here but I don't like the preacher. He doesn't say anything." I nodded to her and then sang.

On a hill far away stood an old rugged cross, the emblem of suffering and shame. The faraway look came over her face again. She didn't speak, but took a deep breath, sighed, and put her head back. I finished three verses of "The Old Rugged Cross," thinking of the last line as I sang it. *And exchange it someday for a crown.* Ruth deserved a crown, I thought.

Without stopping I modulated into another hymn. *When peace like a river attended my way, when sorrows like sea billows roll. Whatever my lot, thou hast taught me to say, even then it is well with my soul.*

Ruth closed her eyes. The only sound, besides my soft singing and the guitar accompaniment, was a crispy rattle from the newspaper sliding from her lap to the floor as her storied hands fell to her sides.

As I hummed a verse of "Amazing Grace," I could see her let her troubles go. She fell asleep and I tiptoed out of the room feeling rather amused at the tenacity of this ancient woman. She was a fighter, and probably had to be.

In contrast to Ruth, my next patient, a petite woman with a fresh hairdo and well-applied lipstick, sat upright in her wheelchair in the sun, looking out the window next to her bed. She was nicely dressed in matching dusty pink sweatpants and sweatshirt, pink anklets folded down in half, and tiny white tennis shoes. The front of her sweatshirt was imprinted with delicate wildflowers in various pastels. I had seen this style shirt elsewhere. It was typical attire for women of that generation.

She looked at me suspiciously when I approached her.

"What a beautiful day isn't it, Lila? You're sitting right there in the sun."

She didn't speak, but continued to stare at me. There was something familiar about her. I was sure I had never given her music before—but maybe I had. It was rare for me to forget a patient encounter; I'd have to look back into my patient notes.

"Lila, would you like some quiet music this afternoon?"

There was still no answer and her eyes seemed to regard me as a threat. Should I stay? I wondered. Something made me persist. I eased up to her, but not as close as I normally came to patients. Leaving space offered her more safety.

In the good old summertime, in the good old summertime. Strolling down the avenue with your baby fine. She moved her eyes away from my face, and began following the motions of my hands playing the guitar.

He'll hold your hand and you'll hold his, and that's a very good sign. You'll be his Tootsie Wootsie in the good old summertime.

A hint of a smile crept out of the corners of her mouth, and a glance at me told me the music had reached her.

"Do you want more music, Lila?" I said. She nodded ever so slightly.

What was it about this woman that caused me to feel so connected to her? She was distant. But there was a familiarity.

Daisy, Daisy give me your answer true. This tune, this favorite of the older folks, reminded me of my Grandma Char who had sat knee to knee with me in another room on this very hall. I sang it to her shortly before she died, a day after her 102nd birthday party.

I'm half-crazy all for the love of you. I envisioned my grandmother as I sang to Lila, this woman all prim and proper, clean and well-coiffed. Both women were well-mannered ladies of their generation. That typical pink sweatshirt with the wildflowers. When I looked more closely I saw little butterflies perched on the faded petals and leaves. And Grandma Char sat there in Lila's wheelchair smiling at me in her reserved way, her delicate hands, like Lila's, resting on her lap, on the dusty pink sweatpants.

Coming back to the present, I left Char and sang for Lila seated in front of me. At that moment I was stunned to finally realize why I was drawn to this silent patient.

Lila was wearing Grandma Char's sweatshirt and sweatpants! If I ventured to look at the name tag on the collar below Lila's hair, I guessed I would have seen Charlotte Duncan Russell written on the iron-on label my cousin painstakingly pressed into our grandmother's clothing when we transferred her to Extended Care.

Lila sat there warmed and beautiful in my grandmother's outfit. I remembered my cousin asking the family if she could donate Char's clothing to the unit after our grandmother's death. A moment of unreality, disorientation floated around me. I was distracted again and felt a little spooked. Char had died only nine months earlier. Her memory, her presence was still fresh. I wanted her to be sitting in the wheelchair in the sun wearing the dusty pink sweatsuit. Not Lila.

I almost asked Lila if she knew she was dressed in a very special person's clothing, to tell her the story of my grandmother and this unusual coincidence. But I stopped myself: Lila was in her own world, not mine.

I sang one more song to her and said a quick good-bye. She didn't wave, or thank me, or change her expression.

She just sat there unfazed, in Grandma Char's outfit with the wildflowers and the butterflies.

~~

The next week I arrived at Extended Care when lunchtime ended and the hallways were crowded. Mobile patients raised and set down walkers with each methodical step as they shuffled back to their rooms after eating in the dining room. Other residents returned via wheelchairs, their palms atop the rubber wheels, pushing forward hand over hand. The faster wheelchair drivers used their feet in a walking motion to propel themselves home. I wondered why they were in such a hurry.

Today there was a traffic jam. A heaped laundry cart and all the patient vehicles clogged the hallway right near Ruth's room. Over all the commotion I heard a loud monologue and recognized a familiar commanding, agitated voice.

"I told them not to seat me next to her. All she does is complain and I don't like it." Ruth was talking to no one in particular.

I squeezed my way through the maze of equipment and people to reach her.

She recognized me as I came closer.

"You know what they did to me today? They sat me next to that woman at lunch. I don't like her and I told them last time not to put me next to her ever again. I'm all upset. She upsets me."

While Ruth ranted, some of the traffic abated and I decided to unfold my chair in front of her right there in the hallway. She clearly needed calming and she wasn't about to stop her loud protests and move on until someone acknowledged her.

I unzipped my instrument case, pulled out my guitar and sang.

Peace is flowing like a river. Flowing out of you and me. Flowing out...

Suddenly Ruth thrust forward in her wheelchair looking directly at my mouth and blurted out, "Are those your own teeth?"

Without skipping a beat I answered, "Yes," and continued *...flowing out into the desert, setting all the captives free.* She interrupted again. "Well, they're beautiful and you better take care of them," she said, then leaned back in her wheelchair. I sang the rest of the song about peace and healing and love. Ruth settled down and completely lost her train of thought, finally wheeling herself into her room.

Probably to read *The New York Times*.

Chapter 22

Five Wishes: "You Think I'm Old and Feeble?"

I didn't expect the MHTP classes to be so relevant, so practical to both my internship and my eventual work as a CMP. Nor did I expect they would play a significant role in my personal life.

During the session on death and dying, the instructor held up a document entitled "Aging with Dignity: Five Wishes." As she passed one out for each of us, she said, "I suggest you read this, keep it on hand, even fill it out for yourselves." Class ended, and nothing more was said. I scanned the pages, then filed the stapled papers away in my notebook.

Memories of the confusion, the uncertainty, the lack of knowledge surrounding my father's illness and eventual death prompted me to dig out and read the document when my mother was preparing to move from Northville, New York into a continuing care residence community in Norfolk, Virginia. I was impressed with its clarity and specificity about end-of-life care and concerns, and I made several copies, one each for my husband and me, and one for my elderly mother. I placed the original copy back in my notebook.

"Mom, I think this would be a good thing to go over together before you move," I said as I handed over her copy of "Five Wishes."

"What? You think I'm getting old and feeble?" she said with a chuckle in her voice. She and I enjoyed joking with each other, especially in difficult times. Her sense of humor was what I appreciated most about her. My own ability to see through the seriousness, and often the craziness of life, with a joke, a gesture, or a pun often rescued tense interactions with my mother and played a major role in every aspect of my life. I employed humor to stay sane.

"Yeah, you've got one foot in the grave," I joked. "I'd be happy to have some of your energy any day of the week!"

I was my mother's only daughter and the one in the family who put issues of life and death on the table. I assumed my forthrightness came from the sudden loss of my first husband in Vietnam, my own serious cancer experience, and now my work in the field with the elderly, the critically ill, and the dying. I could not but know that life was fragile.

"Why don't you read it over first and then we'll sit down together and fill it out?" She agreed and readily discussed it with me; then she had me write in her responses to the very detailed questions probing her desires about care, her life when she was unable to make her own decisions.

"Five Wishes," an addendum to a Living Will, Health Care Proxy, or Durable Power of Attorney, gets right down to the nitty-gritty about comfort and care. I've witnessed families quarrel, even stop speaking to each other over seemingly petty issues about what ought to or ought not to be done when their loved one either hadn't specified her wishes in detail or provided them at all. With such uncertainty, an already befuddled family can make decisions driven by crisis and emotion rather than thoughtfulness or compassion—decisions they may regret later.

In Mom's case, she was sure she wanted personal care like manicures, hair-washing and combing, tooth-brushing, warm baths, gentle massage, hand-holding, soft music, right up to the end—as long as they didn't cause her pain or discomfort. I expected her to want those measures of comfort since she was fastidious about her hygiene and appearance. She didn't like people to see her sick, needy, unkempt, so I was surprised when she said, "I don't want to be alone in the 'end end'."

She also said she wanted to hear religious readings and poetry. I didn't expect that either, and I realized I didn't know her favorite poems or Bible passages. It was a special moment between us when she told me what she loved in the Bible, and of her fondness for many of the old English poets.

The section in "Five Wishes" about what to do after her death allowed me to write down points she wanted made in her obituary, as well as her choices for music and readings for her memorial service. I knew she wanted to be cremated and have her ashes buried next to my father's in the family plot in Northville. There was already a headstone marking the spot.

Mom signed and dated "Five Wishes" in my presence; it was then filed with her important papers. Our time together that day brought us closer, and I gained new insight into my mother from her answers to the "Five Wishes" questions. Since she was moving, she was pleased that it was recognized by all fifty states as a legal and binding document, a nice confirmation that addressing these issues, which raised some difficult realities for her, was worth her time and effort.

Two years after my mother's departure for Norfolk, Gordon and I also left Northville. The romance of the lake house and the small village wore off with the reality of long winters and long trips to amenities, and less extended family around. When we updated our legal documents with an eldercare attorney in our new residence in Asheville, North Carolina, I brought up "Five Wishes," as I did periodically. Gordon resisted. "It's depressing. I don't want to think about that stuff," he said. Like him, many are reluctant to face mortality. Understandable.

"Hon, I know what you want in health, in life. I want to know your desires when you can't express them. And, I want you to know the same for me, "I said.

"Okay, okay," he said, plopping himself down on the sofa. I sensed his discomfort. Forcing the issue had become very important to me. Why tempt fate? Sudden illness, a terrible accident, lingering life, in all these cases the victim's own words and signature helped the family through an already heart-wrenching situation. I didn't want our children or either of us to wrestle with these questions when harsh realities of life and death smacked us in the face.

Filling out our answers and then sharing them prompted some of the best discussions of our long marriage. I wanted only Hospice care, no prolonging of my life if my healthcare providers predicted that my death was to occur within six months. I was surprised that Gordon wanted more measures taken to save or prolong his life. He mentioned he wanted me to consider CPR, intubation, feeding tubes, treatment for terminal illness, to the very end. We both agreed that with advanced Alzheimer's, which we defined as not knowing any person close to us, we didn't want to be treated for an infection or a heart attack or stroke, anything that prolonged life. In that case, no advanced life support or heroics, even for him.

Cremation, scattering of our ashes, music at our services, scripture, poetry, messages to our loved ones. All this information was recorded, neatly signed, sealed, and stored with our legal documents, our lawyer, and with our elder son, who is our executor. We decided to have our copies notarized since some states require it.

I readily spread the word about "Five Wishes" when the topic of aging and end-of-life care comes up in conversation. I am amazed how many people of any age don't know of this well-crafted tool. Even our lawyer wasn't familiar with it.

My elderly Uncle Norm remembered my talking about "Five Wishes" and called me about obtaining a copy when his wife, my dearest Aunt Nan, was rushed to the hospital in serious condition. He didn't use a computer, so ordering the document online was not an option. I mailed him two copies, one for Nan and one for himself.

Amazingly, my aunt improved and eventually went home, well enough to talk about "Five Wishes." They knew they had dodged a bullet with Nan's recovery. "Rob, thanks for the copies. We've had some good talks and already filled out everything. I still have some questions, though. In today's paper I read that a class on 'Five Wishes' is being offered at the adult learning center. I signed up."

He called me when it was over, saying how informative it was. "But I found a loophole," he said.

He told me that if a 911 call was made, the rescue squad would automatically proceed with heroic, life-saving measures unless they were handed a legal document specifying other directives and signed in the victim's own hand. If such documents were already scanned into the hospital's system, they could honor those as well. "I'm calling my local representative; something needs to be done about this." He was eighty-five, and I was astounded about how proactive he had become.

After his call I copied our "Five Wishes" and "'Do Not Resuscitate" orders and put them in an envelope with our list of medications in a drawer by the refrigerator. I also carried them with me to my next doctor's appointment and had them scanned into the hospital system.

The unexpected and startling news in all this occurred when Uncle Norm began coughing up blood not long after Aunt Nan's recovery. He was transported by ambulance to the hospital, where he learned he had a voracious, incurable form of lung disease that was killing him. The only way to remain alive was having oxygen forced into his lungs, which meant living out his days in the hospital ICU, tethered to a special oxygen rig above his bed. The doctor told him there was no way to determine how long he could go on like this.

Uncle Norm and Aunt Nan already knew what the choices for the situation would be. With his family around him, he read what he had written in "Five Wishes" and chose a date and a time when he would cease treatment and go on comfort care. One of his children objected strongly, but Uncle Norm and Aunt Nan stood firm in their decisions, made not in haste but thoughtfully and carefully at a time when there was no emergency pushing them.

Over the next few days every member of Uncle Norm's family—his wife, children, grandchildren, great-grandchildren and their spouses— filed into his hospital room one at a time to sit with him at his bedside, where they exchanged words of comfort, gratitude, and love. Each had a chance to say good-bye.

Just ten days after his diagnosis, on a Saturday evening in early December, the date he chose to cease treatment, my aunt called from the hospital so I could say farewell to my uncle over the phone. He had declined rapidly over the past week and was ready to die with no further suffering, his or his family's. Comfort care was going to start at 7 p.m. when his doctor removed the oxygen.

"Uncle Norm, I respect your decision, but I'll miss you. Your choice is really courageous and compassionate. I'm proud of you. I love you. You've made a difference in my life."

He was able to choke out only two words. "Thanks, Rob."

I hung up the phone and sat stunned at what was actually playing out with my dear Uncle Norm. Doubt took me by surprise. Was this the right thing? Had I influenced him to make this decision? Was this the way life was supposed to end?

Seven o'clock arrived and I pictured my aunt and cousins seated around Norm's bed, holding his hand, stroking his head, talking quietly to him as he released into his own passing. I wished I had been there to offer music. Instead, I held my own prayerful vigil, keeping him close to me even though he was miles away. With no struggle, no pain, no panic his body let go four hours later at 11 p.m.

No one expected he would get his wish so soon.

Uncle Norm planted the seed for making the desires of the ill and dying more available to family, friends, caregivers. Massachusetts, where he lived, and other states now have a policy that addresses his concerns about emergency treatment.

Sometimes we want what we want even if we know it's going to kill us.

—Donna Tartt, *The Goldfinch*

Chapter 23

Choosing to Go Home: A Toast to Life

"Where's Pat?" I asked.

Kathleen looked up from her desk. "Pat's gone home." Then she went back to her paperwork.

Gone home. Kathleen, and Hospice in general, didn't use such euphemisms about death. Unlike the general population, dying was what it was, simply dying. By the time patients and families made the decision to enter into Hospice care, the dancing around the reality of life's final act was usually reckoned with.

"Croaked," "bit the bullet," "bit the dust," "kicked the bucket," "gone to Jesus," "gone to heaven," "passed on," "gone on," "big sleep," "eternal rest"— hundreds of euphemisms for death saturate our culture, even poke fun at it. Death is removed from everyday life and ushered off to hospitals and nursing homes. Hospice eases the situation and uses the term "crossed over," a phrase that I sometimes adopt to lighten my own grief after losing a loved one, a patient, a friend. "Crossing over" sounds gentle and hopeful.

The sound of the word "dead" or "died" rings with finality. The very sound of the last "d" of these words summons the thud of a coffin lid, the power of a shovel against the dirt as it digs a grave. The end. It's all over.

That didn't ring true for me. I was coming to believe, even know that there was some kind of "crossing over." The "d" in dead wasn't final. "Energy is neither created nor destroyed," says the first law of thermodynamics. Einstein later reiterated it. Ashes to ashes, dust to dust, yes, but that's the body, not the soul. A soul's energy lives on. Once created, as the law says, energy is not destroyed. As I worked with more and more dying patients, I thought about these things more frequently.

I learned that Pat, a Hospice resident whose health improved over her nine months at the House, actually returned to her home. Kathleen said Pat would be welcomed back into the Hospice system whenever she needed it again. Although this was unusual, patients left the House to go home for various reasons. Pat got stronger. I knew the extraordinary care of the staff (and maybe my music) helped her regain her health, become well enough to sign out.

Down the Hospice hall from Pat's room I spotted Ernie, a new patient, in a wheelchair. He looked like a gruff old guy and was a notorious resident of Northville. He wheeled himself with determination toward me and the nurses' station. I knew him vaguely. Mostly knew the stories about him.

"If you see that red Chevy on the road, look out. It's Ernie," my cousin warned me when we first relocated to Northville. "Even the kids scatter out of his way," she said.

"Yeah, that's old Ernie," Jane said smiling when I asked her about the man sitting on the bench outside of Stewart's, the local convenience store, day in and day out, smoking one cigarette after the other. He seemed perfectly happy, enjoying his smokes and greeting everyone who frequented the busy store.

"He's really sweet," she said. "Have you seen him hand out money to the kids for ice cream?"

"I'll have to pay more attention."

Jane was born and raised in Northville so she knew Ernie well. "He had a rough childhood and ran away at fourteen. When he came back to finish school he acted tough: smoked, drank, got into fights hanging out with the wrong crowd."

Ernie's hair was slicked back and his eyes were bloodshot, but his most noticeable feature was a large bulbous nose, red and purple with broken blood vessels announcing dwindling oxygen. He wore khaki trousers and a cotton plaid shirt, spotless and neatly pressed, and he was always clean-shaven. I heard he had a wife, but I never saw her.

If Ernie was shopping in the grocery store down the main street from Stewart's, you knew it by his ferocious coughing, which easily overpowered the piped-in '60s music engulfing the aisles.

Now at Hospice for advanced COPD and lung cancer, Ernie, with his oxygen tube streaming from that porous nose back to a tank hitched to his wheelchair, looked up and seemed to recognize me. I stopped to chat.

"Hi, Ernie. I heard you were here at the House," I said, making conversation. I had never spoken to him before except to say "hi" in response to his greeting as I entered Stewart's.

"Yeah, I'm not gonna stay," he said with finality. His hands trembled and his legs jumped up and down. I'd seen that phenomenon in other patients whose bodies were starved for air.

"Where's your room? I could come down and play some music later if you want," I said, passing off his comment about leaving as wishful thinking. He was too sick to go home.

"I'm gettin' outta here this afternoon. They won't let me smoke in this goddamn place," he said. I saw anger redden his face.

"Oh," was all I had to say, rather stunned. COPD, lung cancer, oxygen tank, and now dying. And his only life's pleasure, smoking, was being denied. I understood. Why should he give it up now and endure nicotine withdrawal on top of his other troubles? That's probably why he was so jumpy. It seemed like a cruel policy to inflict on a gravely ill man. I assumed he also missed the social aspect of his smoking. Often I saw other men seated next to him at Stewart's sharing smokes and each other's company.

New York, along with most other states, passed legislation banning smoking at all medical facilities both inside and outside the buildings. Ernie was stuck with the law.

"Well, I could give you some going-home music if you want," I said, still doubting he would be leaving.

"Nah. I'll be outta here soon. I'm not goin' back to that room. I'm just gonna go up and down this hall 'til my ride comes."

"Good luck. I hope you get home," I said and we both moved on.

He was right: he left Hospice that afternoon. When I passed by Stewart's on my way home I saw the red Chevy astride two parking places and Ernie, sitting in his usual spot on the bench, hooked to his portable oxygen, puffing away on a cigarette. No one at Stewart's seemed to mind the open flame warning on his oxygen tank. I think everyone was just glad to see Ernie back in town.

When I first came to the House, patients could smoke on their patios as long as another person was present. That was a reasonable rule, but finding enough personnel to sit with patients as they smoked presented a problem. And often the smoke from their cigarettes drifting inside the House to other patients' rooms created an unpleasant, nauseous odor for the nonsmokers.

When Ann arrived there, she could smoke outside on her patio with a companion. She was a classy woman, in her early eighties, with perfectly styled hair and expensive clothing. Kathleen told me Ann was from old money earned in the heyday of the glove industry. She inherited a large Victorian home on an expansive manicured lot in the best part of town in Gloversville. At first she still played golf and bridge at the country club and enjoyed lunches out with friends. I was never quite sure why she chose to come to Hospice House. She was a private person and I never asked. It seemed invasive even to ask Kathleen.

Ann accepted my offers of playing and singing for her, but never really engaged in the music. She was restless and distracted. On nice days, she'd suggest we go outside on her patio for the music. And then she'd light up a cigarette. Often the breeze blew the smoke my way, and my singing soon gave way to coughing. This didn't faze her in the least. But it did me.

As winter approached and outdoor temperatures dipped, she'd bundle herself up in one of her expensive coats and request we go outside for music.

"No, I can't take my instruments out in the cold," I told her. I knew I was being used as a cigarette monitor, but avoided making a scene about her smoking. I wasn't a fan of it myself, but that didn't mean she had no right to smoke. Anyway, I was the House musician, not a smoking companion. She'd just have to find another volunteer.

After that she rarely wanted music. I stuck my head in her door more than once to find her out on her patio, oxygen tube removed and lying across her bed, violating the Hospice policy about smoking alone.

Kathleen and the whole staff knew it. They stretched the rules to honor patients' needs.

I happened to stay late at Hospice one afternoon. I saw Ann's elbows parked on the nurses' station counter. She was talking to the nurse on duty. It was four-thirty.

"It's almost five o'clock, why can't I have it now?"

"Your doctor's given written orders for five o'clock," the nurse said.

"Oh, c'mon. It won't hurt if it's early," Ann pleaded.

"I'm sorry, but you'll have to wait."

Ann snorted, turned around with her walker, and mumbled down the hall toward her room.

"What's that about?" I asked.

"Ann's medication orders include two martinis a day at 5 p.m."

"You're kidding!" I laughed.

"Nope. The gin and vermouth are locked up right there in the meds closet," she said pointing to the door where all the patient medications were kept behind a secure, coded entry. "And those bottles go down fast. She likes a stiff drink. We're always ordering her booze from the liquor store."

I shook my head in amazement. "Two martinis, and stiff ones at that."

"It's actually a pain. After she drinks we have to watch her. She gets a little tipsy and she can fall."

"I'm surprised this is allowed."

"Luckily she eats her dinner after her cocktails, and goes right to bed, around six-thirty."

"Does anyone else have alcohol on their meds chart?" I asked.

"Only Ann. She tries to finagle a drink out of us other times of the day, too. It's a problem," she stated, busying herself with a pen and clipboard.

I wanted to know more, but I probably already knew more than I really needed to know. HIPAA and MHTP classes taught that we should inquire only about what was needed to perform our specified duties. Ann's alcoholic medication fell out of that sphere.

The next time I saw Ann she was talking on the phone in her room. She glanced up and motioned for me to come in. I walked in with my guitar and sat in one of her upholstered side chairs, enjoying how beautifully decorated her room was. Her own furniture and appointments erased any thoughts of a Hospice patient residing there. The only signs of infirmity were the oxygen concentrator groaning off to the side of her bed, the clear plastic tube running from it to Ann's nostrils, and the polished silver walker in the corner by her bed.

She hung up the phone and spoke. "I'm calling around to some apartments in Saratoga to see when they'll have openings."

"Are you planning to move out of the House?"

"Yes. I don't think I need the care here," she said. "They don't let me live my life."

"Will you hire a caregiver if you go out on your own?" I asked.

"I have a friend who knows someone who'll get my meals and do housework."

"Will she stay with you all the time?" I was concerned about Ann's safety, her medical needs.

"She'll go home after dinner."

"Will you be safe all night on your own?"

"I sleep all night. I'm sure I'll be fine. I think I'll be happier."

I sat there in disbelief. Ann was serious about moving to an apartment. But she was right: her lifestyle was compromised at Hospice. She knew the new state law about smoking was about to take effect, and already she was unable to enjoy her cocktails. I hoped a new diagnosis had not also prompted her decision.

"I wish you well with your search. Saratoga ought to have some very nice living options," I said, feeling sad for this proud but vulnerable woman. "Oh, and do you want music today?"

"I just wanted to tell you I'm leaving."

"Thanks. I'll keep up with your progress," I said rising from the chair and stepping toward the door. The thought of Ann being on her own didn't sit well with me, but I was touched that she thought to tell me about her plans.

We waved good-bye and I left her as she picked up the phone again and directed her attention to the Yellow Pages open on her lap.

I knew why Ann was leaving—and it wasn't about a nicer place to live or better care. It was about freedom.

She ought to recapture it while she could, I thought.

When I got outside her room, I smiled thinking about the martinis. She would definitely be sleeping through the night.

The whole drift of my education goes to persuade me that the world of our present consciousness is only one out of many worlds of consciousness that exist, and that those other worlds must contain experiences which have meaning for our life also... The two become continuous at certain points, and higher energies filter in.

—William James, *Varieties of Religious Experience*

Chapter 24

Staying in the Mystery

No one had actually died in my presence over the several months I had been providing music at bedsides. I had been expecting it with so many patients, had practiced the protocol for the actively dying, had seen the MHTP training go to work. I wasn't fearful of death. I think I was more curious than anything. Even my own dad had died without me, just two rooms away in our house. When other CMPs spoke of their experiences with patients' actual passing, I felt like I was missing the full range of what I had to offer and learn from the experience.

When Kathleen directed me to Walter, an elderly patient I'd never met before, I was relieved that I was prepared. He had all the signs of imminent death: Cheyne-Stokes breathing, mottled hands and feet, pale skin, closed eyes, and pure non-responsiveness. At any second his family, gathered around his bed at the House, and I, settled next to him on my chair with my harp, expected the next exhalation to be his last.

Playing irregular beats, following Walter's spotty inhales and exhales with the long spaces after each breath, a random chord or note here, a small run of the notes there, fully disconnected. Low notes on the harp. Minor key if you could even call it a key. This process took much anticipation and heavy concentration. And it felt stilted.

I wondered what his relatives thought of this technique. They may have had similar thoughts as I once did about playing a person's favorite music as he died. It would have been a lot easier for me to do this, but there I was plucking randomly, feeling like I was nearly dying with Walter myself, my respiration matching his just as the music did.

No one seemed to pay much attention to the music. The family was well dressed, dignified, with respect for the expertise of the Hospice staff. I could see that included me. Men in business suits and ties. Women in heels and hose, nicely coiffed, good jewelry. Now and then one of them stepped to the hallway and made a call, keeping their talking brief and to a whisper. Staff had probably told them that the dying can hear up until the very end.

Muted light illumined Walter's room. No photos or cards or flowers or food lay around his room. From these clues I assumed he had not been at the House very long.

It must have been thirty or forty-five minutes that I gently plucked the harp strings matching Walter's fading breaths. The silences between exhales and inhales became longer. Kathleen periodically slipped in to the room to check on him. There were no moistened lollipop sponges swabbed around his lips. I guessed at this stage he could choke on the tiniest drop of water, an awful way to die. He was so close.

Besides listening to respirations, I watched Walter's chest, the only part of his body still moving. In fact, his breathing became so shallow, so silent, that his chest was my only guide.

And then his chest finally stopped moving.

But I didn't stop playing. Something led me to continue. I slightly picked up the beat and started playing unobtrusively, softly, and with recognizable music. Melodic, beautiful soulful and rhythmic music. Something about Walter's body was bidding me to play on.

Kathleen entered the room to listen to Walter's heart and nodded to the gathered family that he had finally passed. She glanced at her watch and recorded the time of death. She would be responsible for filling out the death certificate. No one burst into tears, or grabbed a cell phone to report the news. Walter died but no one moved a muscle as I continued with the music.

The Hospice nurses in my classes had shared post-mortem experiences that intrigued me. They said rather casually that with many patients, they saw a white light or sensed a hovering presence above the patient's body immediately after death. I wondered whether I would ever experience this phenomenon.

I certainly couldn't account for staying put, playing for Walter after his death. I did intensely feel there was something ethereal in the room, a whitish glow hovering above Walter's still body. Was it just the light from the window? It seemed to be hanging close to him, a real part of him, unable to let go, almost asking permission to leave him. Was this what my nurse friends meant?

I played on, mesmerized by what I came to believe was a holy presence. I think the music went on for close to fifteen minutes. Time and space vanished. Walter's family must have felt the sanctity of the moment as well. I noticed they were holding hands, circled around his bed. And I heard some quiet crying in the background of the harp music.

Was this Walter's soul, his true essence stationed above him? Or was this presence beckoning Walter's soul to leave his body? Were they merging?

I finally felt the urge to stop playing. I think that's when Walter's soul finally left his body. Heads turned toward me in the new silence. We made eye contact. I think his family knew we had experienced a holy moment and that Walter had really crossed over now. A middle-aged man from the family stepped into the hallway and made a call on his phone. Others in the room began talking quietly among themselves. I slowly and methodically removed myself and my chair from the private space, carrying my precious harp under my arm.

On the way out of the room I stopped at the end of Walter's bed and whispered, "Blessings, Walter. And blessings all the way around."

I hoped no staff was in the hall. I didn't want to talk. What had happened? What had just held me in its arms, revealed itself? I wanted to keep it there, extend the sacredness, the full heart, the expanded spirit resting in me. I walked to the Serenity Room at the end of the hallway, quietly letting myself in and closing the door behind me. Trying to make sense of things, I lowered myself on to the sofa, inhaled, and put my head back to look toward heaven.

Heaven. Is there really a heaven, an afterlife? Did I just witness ascendance to heaven, the beautiful and hushed crossing over from life to death? Or was it life to more life? Energy merged with energy?

White light. So much about white light in near-death accounts. Now I saw white light with an actual death. When I was severely ill with cancer treatment and terrified I would die, a white light hovered over me one dark night and a voice filled my head saying, "You don't need to be afraid. I'm taking care of you." Was this the same kind of light that hovered above Walter? Could this be a form of God?

Healers I've worked with, over the course of both physical and emotional illnesses in my life, helped me visualize white light as healing energy. I think it's the same prayerful essence I call forth when I enter a patient's room, picturing the doorway encircled with the energy, the spirit, the love I need to offer healing music to the ill and dying.

As I rested and contemplated what I had just experienced, I felt comforted. I wasn't in charge of any of it, and I don't believe the music summoned it. I was merely led to follow what was already there. The music allowed me and Walter's family to stay present for it.

Like Walter, other patients have blessed me with their ascensions. The phenomenon is unpredictable but similar every time. There is something to this white light. I can say for sure that my own belief about an afterlife has taken root. And I have been privy to unexplained healings as well.

I am humbled to think I am one such healer. I can't explain it. It comes unexpectedly. And therein lies its beauty, its power, its mystery.

~~

Good music creates an intersection between heaven and the soul.

—Aniekee Tochukwu

Psychology of Friendship for Leadership, 2010

Chapter 25

Playing in the Key of G

I thought I'd be ready when she died. More ready than most. By this time I had offered music as a CMP to so many infirmed, elderly, and dying people, and I had been present several times at the moment of death.

But I was wrong.

This patient was my mother.

Her love was complicated. I danced all my life for her to show me, tell me, that she loved me. For her to notice me, appreciate me, especially as a musician. She expected much, criticized much. I blamed it on her New England upbringing, her unusual childhood. But I still yearned for her affection, and her approval.

My life was riddled with stories of disappointing my mother despite my best efforts. I remember eagerly bounding down from the junior high auditorium stage where, as a seventh grader, I had just taken a bow after flawlessly performing a difficult violin solo by memory. I slid into my seat in the audience next to her. The full house was still clapping for my accomplishment when I looked to her for her response. When the applause died down, she bent over to me and whispered, "Robin, you stood up there like a farmer."

My heart stopped. I knew what she meant. Suddenly I felt ashamed of my big feet, my height, my athletic frame. I was wearing the dark red dress with the ruffles on the hem and sleeves, the one she chose for me, but that wasn't enough. I wasn't the petite, frilly daughter she wanted up there on stage. Ironically, planting my feet while standing and playing violin was one of the first lessons my teacher taught me.

My mother and I shared music together, but for many years we were on different ends of the music spectrum. She, a classically trained vocalist and pianist with her music degree, me with some classical training, but mostly a free spirit, playing by ear, improvising, embracing music with voice and multiple instruments across genres.

As a high school student enamored with the emerging sixties folk scene, I latched onto the music of Ian and Sylvia, marveling at their unique style, their delicious vocal harmonies, the energy of Ian's guitar; I played their records full blast on my father's stereo in our living room. I made sure no one, especially my mother, was home. One afternoon, while my favorite "Early Morning Rain" filled the house, she arrived early and heard me singing my lungs out.

"Robin, turn that off. That music is terrible. They can't sing. Hear how they sustain their notes on consonants? You never do that. You sustain on vowels. Don't ever sing like that."

I continued to sing and learn to play instruments, my way. I also continued to perform and enjoy classical music, her way. Like her, I gave private music lessons. Unlike hers in the middle of the living room, I gave students lessons on guitar and dulcimer in my private home studio, which Gordon and I built so that normal life could go on despite the presence of students in our home.

I hired baby sitters to tend our children. Her lesson-giving dominated our family life. I was forbidden to invite friends over after school on her lesson days, four days a week. On those days I had to come straight home to babysit my brothers and put dinner in the oven. Those responsibilities followed me through grade school and middle school.

Not until I performed and recorded multiple CDs of folk and old-timey music with the Mill Run Dulcimer Band in the 1980s did she consider my kind of music legitimate, and me a real musician. She and my father were regulars at the Band concerts, and I think my being a performer on stage gave her bragging rights. She depended on me to provide her with a list of my accomplishments for her annual Christmas letter to friends and family.

Even then, she never stopped teaching me—or correcting me. It seemed she never really recognized my musical gifts. According to her, using printed music, reading notes was what real musicians did: I wondered if she was jealous that I could effortlessly play by ear, transpose, improvise.

Do, a deer, a female deer; re, a drop of golden sun; mi, a name I call myself... I sang with enthusiasm as she lay bedridden but awake and aware just two weeks before she died. *The Sound of Music* had been a family favorite; we knew all the songs.

"Robin, that's *do, sol, mi, re,* on the last line. You're singing it *do, do, do, do.*"

"Oh, okay." I knew I was singing do, oh, oh, oh, but I didn't argue with my mother when it came to music. In fact, I didn't argue with her about much of anything. She always got the last word. I resumed singing.

My shepherd will supply my need, Jehovah is His name. In pastures fresh He makes me feed beside the living stream. This moving, musical setting of the "The Twenty-Third Psalm" was a favorite for both of us. I looked to her for some recognition as I sang it, some meeting of our eyes, maybe even some tears, but instead she spoke when I ended.

"Robin, I want you to sing 'Do, Re, Mi' again so I know you've got it right." I smiled, complied. Just as I always had.

From her surgery eight months earlier, until this time, I played and sang my heart out to her during each visit we made to Harbor's Edge, her classy Continuing Care Retirement Community in Norfolk. During those months, with mounting physical infirmities, she bounced between the hospital, her apartment, and the healthcare floors of Harbor's Edge.

During Easter I brought the blue Presbyterian hymnal that contained the music she knew so well from her days as a music minister. "Would you like to sing some of the Easter music, Mom?"

"I'm not sure I can sing very well but I'd like to hear it. Sure," she said, looking away.

I opened the hymnal to the Easter section and began with the first song, accompanying myself on the Goya. I needed the book for the words. *Christ is risen! Shout Hosannah! Celebrate this day of days!* I sang all the way through while she watched; I knew I was being scrutinized again.

"You know, Robin, that's the tune to 'Ode to Joy' by Beethoven. I hope you played it in the key of G. That's the right key."

"Yes, I did, but I can play it in any key!" I may have said that to get a rise out of her.

"But you don't do that. It was written in the key of G."

She knew the key signature of every hymn and became annoyed if I transposed from what was written. "That's always in E flat," she said when I sang "Thine Is the Glory."

"E flat is not a great key for guitar unless I have a capo." Why did I even bother to say it?

For most of the music I gave her, she seemed preoccupied when I sang and played. She fumbled with her clothes, read mail, stared away from me, picked at her forehead, adjusted her bedcovers, asked for water or ice, watched the clock. I didn't expect it. Nor did I like it.

I was trying so hard to love her, to reach her, to connect with her. The love in my music was open, honest, direct. How could she miss it? Maybe she didn't want to see herself as a patient, my patient, in need of healing. Maybe she felt controlled. Maybe she felt overwhelmed. Maybe she was afraid. Or maybe I was right: she simply did not consider me a real musician.

But then, after the session of music with "Do, Re, Mi," even with my "mistake," she surprised me with an unexpected, and unlooked-for, compliment.

"I really enjoyed that, Robin," she said. Her words were a gift from heaven, a glimpse of her complicated love.

~~

My mother's health continued to decline and baffle the doctors. I knew she was going seriously downhill when she no longer reacted to my interjections of humor. I could usually make her laugh through the most unbearable, tense moments. We enjoyed that connection together. Now even this was gone, and the distance between us widened. Finally she was diagnosed with end-stage renal failure. Ironic. The same disease Dad had died of, twelve years before.

Calls between me and Hospice and her bedside caregiver grew in intensity and frequency.

"Is it time to come? Is she in transition?" I'd ask. She had written in her "Five Wishes" that she wanted a family member with her for the "end end" as she called it. I wanted to be that person.

"It's hard to say; her vitals are strong but she's certainly declining," the Hospice nurse said more than once. "But, I don't think she's going to die by the book," she added.

"That would be my mother," I said.

When the private caregiver gave me an updated report by phone, saying that Mom was clamping her lips shut, refusing food and drink, even her favorite hot tea, I knew things had changed. It felt as though the "end end" was approaching.

Gordon and I threw things in the car and took off midafternoon. While he drove, I made phone calls to relatives and friends alerting them to Mom's sure decline and probable passing. "You might want to call and say good-bye tomorrow when we're here to pick up the phone," I said. "We'll be by her side until we take a lunch break. It might help her to hear you one last time."

I thought about how, after my cousin's and middle brother's visits just two days earlier, Mom began to let go. I smiled thinking she might have been waiting for them—and actually was doing something by the book.

As the miles ticked away I became more nervous about how she would look when we finally arrived. My adrenaline surged when I pushed her door open and crept into her room.

The oxygen concentrator clicked and hissed. The room was dark except for the glow of the little stained glass lamp I had placed on her dresser when she was moved to the Skilled Care floor—the lamp I had given her ten years ago for her eightieth birthday. She took in easy breaths through her mouth, toothless and gaping open. Seeing her without her teeth was rare and hard. It had always frightened me. This time I took it in stride.

I walked over to her bed and leaned close to her good ear. "Hi, Mom. It's Robin. Gordon and I are here." I smoothed her forehead, kissed her, and took her hand. She didn't respond.

"Mom, it's Robin. We're here," I said hoping for some sign she heard me.

Again there was no response, so I sat down next to her, still and silent, caressing her hand. The dim room, her warm thin body, her soft pink floral knit nightgown, the family photos and memorabilia neatly placed so she could see them, gave me a sense of peace. She was well cared for, and I knew I had done my part to ensure that. Each of her desires in "Five Wishes" had been granted. I recalled the remark she often made when Gordon and I came to town to tend her: "Robin, when you come, things really get done." I hoped I could do something now.

My brother Glenn, who lived in Norfolk, was taking care of her business affairs and stopping in to see her around his work schedule. Both my other brothers worked full-time and lived out of town. We all did what we could.

I remembered how Gordon and I would tell her we were heading back to Asheville after our visits with her. I'd say, probably out of guilt, "Mom, I know you hate to see us go, but we need to get back home." She'd reply, "Yes, who wouldn't. You spoil me." That statement, perhaps an indirect way of saying "Thanks" or "I love you," made me feel good. At least she noticed my efforts. Although I had been in counseling on and off for several years, trying to break myself of the need for her approval, I still begged for it in so many ways. Did she think I was a real musician now that I was playing and singing as a CMP? I knew I was doing the right thing by her, being a good daughter, helping my mother die well, and the urgency of her needs held sway over any lingering desire for her to openly love me.

It was now midnight and I was drooping with fatigue. Gordon had already turned in; he had insisted on driving the whole way over.

"Good night, Mom. I'll be back in the morning," I said, gently sliding my hand out of hers, and kissing her on the cheek. I would bring the harp in the morning and play for her.

The next morning she lay in the same position in her bed, her mouth still agape and her teeth out. I nestled down next to her and said, "Good morning, Mom. It's Robin."

"She's pretty sleepy," the caregiver said. "And she won't let me put in her teeth or swab her mouth or lips with the sponges. She just clamps her jaw shut. Her lips are so dry from mouth breathing." This was my first meeting with Mom's private caregiver, my eyes and ears, the person who gave me detailed reports when I called, sometimes multiple times a day.

I could see the caked saliva and dry peeling skin on Mom's lips from lack of hydration. "Maybe she'd allow you to put Vaseline on her lips," I said. The caregiver agreed. "I'll try to find some," she said and disappeared out the door. I set up my harp and began playing, then singing with the accompaniment.

Oh, Danny boy, the pipes, the pipes are calling; from glen to glen and down the mountainside. She liked the sweeping arpeggios of my playing and usually sang with me on this song.

"Mom," I said, hoping for a glimmer of a response, "remember you played your favorite arrangement of 'Danny Boy' on St. Patrick's Day?"

Playing the piano was at the top of her bucket list. On St. Patrick's Day, just five weeks earlier, I had encouraged her to play, helped her shuffle behind her walker to the piano in her apartment, eased her to the bench and stood close behind her as her frail, inexact fingers tried to find the right notes. Before her illness, she performed regular solo piano concerts at Harbors Edge.

"I need to practice. My hands are so weak," she said, stopping and shaking her head.

"Mom, this arrangement is so beautiful. I'd like to hear all of it."

She struggled her way to the end of the music, granting my wish. My intention in coaxing her was for her to fulfill her own wish, but she may have been too sick to care at that point. It was hard to read her. Was she merely pleasing me?

Now even with my playing and singing "Danny Boy," she didn't open her eyes or move her lips. I continued playing more melodic Irish music, then put down the harp and began to sing. She was restful and calm. Rather than take up my guitar, I sang a cappella to her so I could hold her hand and lean down close to her ear. I put my cheek next to hers, feeling how baby-soft and warm it was. I hoped the vibration of my voice through her body might resonate in some deep place in her.

"Mom, can you squeeze my hand if you'd like to hear 'The Trumpet Vine'?" This song was another favorite. Its lyrics spoke of friendship and relationship. I wondered why it spoke to her. I felt her fingers faintly tighten against my hand. *The trumpet vine grew in the kitchen window and bloomed bright orange on the wall; you sat in the morning light holding a guitar as the first summer rains began to fall.* I saw a tiny tear well up in her left eye.

"Oh, look she's crying," said the caregiver who had returned with Vaseline and was watching Mom closely as she had for several weeks.

"This is a special song for her." My parents had loved me singing the lead with the Mill Run Dulcimer Band; the song was my first recorded solo. It always made Dad cry, and of course I'd sung it at his memorial service. I was surprised I could get through it now.

"Mom, can you squeeze again if you'd like to hear 'Roseville Fair'?"

Again, a faint squeeze.

Oh, the night was clear and the stars were shining, and the moon came out so quiet in the sky. And the people gathered round and the band was a tunin', I can hear them now playin', "Coming Through the Rye."

Her face looked so smooth, even young again.

You were dressed in blue and you looked so lovely; just a simple flower of a small-town girl. And you took my hand and we danced to the music, and I made you mine at the Roseville Fair.

She often requested this song, another Band favorite, and I imagined that these lyrics brought back memories of her and my father's courtship. He was smitten by her pure blue eyes, and they loved to slow-dance cheek to cheek. As children, my brothers and I giggled when they danced in our living room as the radio played one of "their" songs.

As I finished the chorus of "Roseville Fair" the phone rang next to her bed. She didn't stir.

"Mom, it's Adam," I said leaning in close to her ear, then holding the phone down to her ear so she could hear her oldest grandchild's words. It was sublime as all her grandchildren and other family members made calls to her that morning. I watched her as they each said their private good-byes. I took back the phone when I could tell they were finished speaking, and reported what I thought might have been some responses from her. "She moved her lips after you spoke," I said. "It looked to me like she was trying to say 'I love you' or maybe 'thank you'." I'd noted over the years how it was easier for her to be openly expressive with her grandchildren than with me or my brothers.

I resumed singing song after song to her, all familiar music. Occasionally her mouth closed and a pencil-thin line appeared across her lips. Was she smiling? Maybe she was present in some way for the music I was offering. Between songs I petted her face, massaged her hand, spoke softly to her.

"Mom, we kids are all adults now," I said. "We'll take care of each other and our families. We don't want you to suffer anymore. I love you." Hospice reminded me and my brothers to tell her this, and to repeat it often either in person or by phone.

Late in the afternoon she required hygienic care. I assisted the nurses holding her up on one side and then the other. With her eyes still closed, she moaned and winced, despite the recent administration of a small dose of liquid morphine. Interestingly, she opened her mouth for the dropper to insert the medicine under her tongue.

"Mom, I know this hurts. It'll be over soon," I said and stroked her forehead with my free hand. It pained me to see her in such misery being touched and manipulated. When the nurses adjusted her nightgown, she suddenly opened her eyes wide and looked straight up at me with surprise, delight. "Robin, you're here," she whispered in a strained voice, smiling at me the whole time.

Stunned, I said, "Yes, Mama. I'm here just as I said I would be." She closed her eyes again and rested back into her pillow as the nurses pulled the sheet up over her. She couldn't stand even the weight of a blanket on her skin.

That smile, those eyes, that greeting. Had it really happened? Was this the "I love you" I had waited for all my life? I replayed it in my head several times, trying to make it so.

The following morning, I opened the music for her with "Danny Boy" on the harp. She became restless, agitated: her feet twitched, her hands clutched the sheet, her face scrunched into a frown. The familiar music, the beat, the same arpeggios on the harp she usually loved were too much for her now. I quickly changed my playing to arrhythmic, melody-free, word-free, low-toned music, the protocol for the actively dying that I had used so successfully with other patients in her state. As her breathing became more shallow and irregular I matched her respirations with an easy ebb and flow of the music.

I wanted to hold her hand again, so I passed the harp over to Gordon and switched the music to improvisational chanting using vowel sounds, *aaaaaah, ohhhhhh, oooooooh*, adding easy consonants with long pauses and no recognizable melody or rhythm in the phrases. Occasionally she moaned, coughed, gurgled. The morphine dosage had been increased to every hour now, but it wasn't enough. Only when I chanted did her struggling cease.

I glanced at Gordon, who sat nearby observing me in my element, both as therapeutic musician and as daughter, helping my mother find her way to the place she believed she was going. "I can't wait to get to heaven and see your father and my father," she had said more than once over the months as her illness diminished her. Gordon saw firsthand how the music calmed her, brought her peace, eased her pain, and in this moment, ferried her along the route to the heaven she was waiting for.

All at once her breathing stumbled. We both stood up over her. I stopped chanting.

She opened her eyes and looked up. Her lips tried to say something. Then she exhaled her last breath and let go. A familiar glow of holy presence engulfed the room.

Then I burst into sobbing, fell across her body and embraced her. "Mama," I cried. "I won't be able to hug you anymore."

Gordon leaned over and held me, stroking my back and shoulders as they heaved with this sudden outburst. I was surprised at my reaction. I wasn't ready.

But in that moment I was no longer a therapeutic musician.

I was only her daughter.

Epilogue

KALANCHOE

In the window,
   two plants—
   Kalanchoe I chose myself.
One for me,
   the other, my mother's.
A sweet blooming pink,
   her color,
   like the nightgown
   I gave her.
She gushed
   when I told her,
   on purpose,
   knowing how she was,
"It's from the Biltmore."

My plant, the red one,
   my color,
   too much for her,
   as always.
I kept it at home
   although she could guess
   which color I chose.
"You've always liked red."
Red cowboy boots,
   the final straw.

The plants dropped their blooms,
   both in my window now
   looking alike.
I lost track.
   Which pink?
   Which red?
Nine stems rose
   out of one,
   surely my red;
   One stem from the other,
   a sign, a holding back
   like always.

December came,
   the first one
   without her;
And nine stems blossomed.

I want to think
She loved me.

Robin Russell Gaiser
February 2015

Discussion Questions

Chapter 1–Throw Me in for One Last Dip

1. What is the purpose of the chapter? Is it only background?
2. How do the setting and the characters relate to each other?
3. What tensions are expressed? By whom? About what?
4. What does the author learn? What do you learn?

Chapter 2 – Is This Music Program a Hoax?

1. How did the author react after her father's death? Have your responses to death been similar or dissimilar?
2. Has someone's death led you to change your own life?
3. There are instances in this chapter that can be seen as coincidences. What are they? What are your thoughts about such occurences?
4. What do you learn about Certified Music Practitioners in this chapter? Had you heard of this form of caregiving before?

Chapter 3 – Welcome to Hospice House

1. Why does the author describe Hospice House in such great detail? Is this what you would expect such a facility to look like?
2. Describe any Hospice experience you have had. What was your reaction? Was it different from what you expected? How? Did the experience change you in any way?
3. The author begins to see the music she offers as ministry. How do you see it?
4. CMP music is patient-centered, a service not a performance. Is that always true?
5. What won Bob over? What changed for him, his family, the author?

Chapter 4 – Almost Heaven—Lavender and Camo

1. What stands out about the surroundings, the characters, the patients in this chapter? What roles do they play?

2. Despite the differences, is there any common ground among them?

3. Does the author employ other roles besides that of a music practitioner? What are they? Are they necessary? Helpful? If so, in what way, and to whom?

4. How does the title of this chapter, "Almost Heaven," apply?

Chapter 5 – Finding My Musical Niche

1. What about the author's background contributes to her decision to become a CMP? (The book's introduction also addresses this question).

2. Differences in making music are presented in this chapter. What are they? Is one style preferable over the other for being a therapeutic musician? How does the quotation from "Let It Be Wild" impact these questions?

3. Can the author's style of music-making be taught?

Chapter 6 – Never Saw a Wolf

1. When Len hesitates about having live music, he finally says, "I like country music. Guitar." Why did he change his tune?

2. Think of the phrase, "playing music." How does this apply to the author and Len?

3. The author expresses concern about doing harm to Len. Did she cause him harm? Why or why not?

4. How does careful listening play a role in this chapter? Is listening done only with the ears?

Chapter 7 – Musical Morphine

1. Where DOES the word "heaven" appear in this chapter? Is it also implied? Where?

2. The author describes patients in graphic detail. Is this necessary? Why or why not?

3. Part of the title of the book originates in this chapter. The author added the subtitle, "Transforming Pain One Note at a Time." Why do you think this was done?

4. Discomfort and awkwardness in the presence of seriously ill or dying persons is a common reaction. Why? The author feels fortunate to have her gift of music to offer in these situations. What special interest or gift could you offer?

Chapter 8 – Kurt Flies Away

1. What voice or voices did Kurt find? How did this affect Kurt?
2. Kurt and the author discover musical similarities. What are they?
3. What different roles does the author play? Do the varying roles serve the same purpose?
4. In what way does music become a character in this chapter? How do the music and Kurt's health mirror each other?

Chapter 9 – Dealer's Choice

1. Compare the hospital extended care facility with Hospice House. What is your reaction to each one?
2. The author realizes she knows very little about Helen. But Helen wants to know about the author. Is it a good idea to form a relationship with a patient? Why or why not?
3. How would you describe Linda Raines? Is she well suited to this job? Why or why not?
4. The author wrestles with being paid for work and volunteering services as a music practitioner. Does either position harm or benefit the other?

Chapter 10 – "One, Two, Three Strikes You're Out"

1. What risks does a therapeutic musician take?
2. What went wrong in this chapter? Is anyone to blame?
3. What does the author learn from this experience?

Chapter 11 – Music: 01, Meds: 00

1. What range of emotions is expressed in this chapter? Which ones stirred you and why?

2. What is wrong or right about this situation? Could or can things be done differently?

3. Who was responsible for making things better for this patient?

4. What does the quotation from *Being Mortal* suggest in response to these issues?

Chapter 12 – Parking My Ego

1. The author approaches this chapter differently. Why?

2. What new information did you learn about the author? How does it enlarge the story?

3. Does this chapter really offer a break? Why or why not?

Chapter 13 – Holding the Music in Her Hands

1. What senses are utilized in this chapter? How do they function?

2. What rules does the author follow? Does observing rules help or hamper patient care? Why?

3. Did Lillian actually hear? What did the nurses think? Why might they think this?

Chapter 14 – Semper Fi

1. What drew the author to engage with Ron?

2. Was there benefit derived from the encounter?

3. Did the author violate Ron's wishes for no music?

Chapter 15 – Deathly Afraid

1. What different story lines occur in this chapter?

2. Peggy's experience was not the norm at Hospice. What was unusual?

3. What other aspects of music practitioner work come to light in this chapter?

4. What interventions did the author employ with Peggy? Did any of these in particular work better than the others? Which one and why?

5. The idea of self-care is introduced in this chapter. Do some jobs or duties require more self-care than others? Which ones, and why? How do you take care of yourself?

Chapter 16 – Pachelbel and Patsy Cline

1. What did you take away from this chapter about food for the very ill and the dying? How will you use this information?
2. Food and music work together in this chapter. How?
3. Why does Sheila eat?
4. What more do you learn about Kathleen, the head nurse at Hospice? What characteristics make her suitable for this job?

Chapter 17 – Last Words

1. What different expressions of "last words" occur in this chapter? To whom are they valuable?
2. Do you have a story about the function of "last words" in your own life?
3. Do "last words" need to be last? Why or why not?
4. Do you agree with the author's statement that "there are no second chances for the living or dying to express last words"?

Chapter 18 – Lost

1. What is your experience with cognitively impaired persons? Have you observed them reacting to music? What was the reaction? How do you react when you hear music from your past?
2. How do these anecdotes illustrate the sweet and heartbreaking sides of cognitive impairment?
3. In what way do you think you would have reacted to the actions of Dave and to the woman rocking her baby doll? Would you go back to their rooms after these incidents? Why or why not?
4. Should MHTP students receive information about these possibilities as part of the curriculum?

Chapter 19 – The Guessing Game

1. Why is singing and playing religious music to patients an issue?
2. Compare Addie's and Hillie's situations. What was the same? What was different?
3. Did the author offer music appropriately to each patient? Why or why not?
4. This chapter adds more information about hospice. What have you learned thus far?

Chapter 20 – Chaos and Clarity

1. Does the author's personal story of cancer add to or take away from Grace's story?
2. Sound plays a starring role in this chapter. How? What do you learn?
3. What clarity comes to light in this chapter? For whom and how?
4. Who paid the author for her memorial service music? Are you sure? Why?

Chapter 21 – Teeth and a Sweatshirt

1. Ruth and Lila are both at extended care. How are they alike? Different?
2. What emotions does each story conjure up for you?
3. How would you describe the tone of this chapter? How does it differ from most of the others?

Chapter 22 – "Five Wishes": Do You Think I'm Old and Feeble?

1. Were you aware of the "Five Wishes" document or ones similar to it before reading this chapter? Are you inclined to study such a document and fill it out? Why or why not?
2. How is such an instrument valuable? To or for whom?
3. Do you agree with Uncle Norm's decision to terminate treatment? What would you do under similar circumstances? How would your family and friends react?
4. Has your state provided means to close the emergency care loophole that Uncle Norm discovered? Why or why not is this a concern?

Chapter 23 – Choosing to Go Home: A Toast to Life

1. The author opens discussion about an afterlife. How would you describe her approach?

2. Doctors, along with the patient and family, make the decision for admission to Hospice. Why did Pat, Ernie, and Ann choose to leave the Hospice House? Was this a sound idea? Why or why not?

3. Do laws and rules governing medical facilities need to be amended for dying patients? Why or why not?

Chapter 24 – Staying in the Mystery

1. What additional ideas about death and afterlife does the author offer after experiencing Walter's death? Have you observed, experienced, or pondered anything similar to what she describes?

2. What does the term "white light" bring to mind? In what contexts is it mentioned in this chapter?

3. The author asks if the light, the essence she sees, may be a form of God. What is your response to that supposition?

Chapter 25 – Playing in the Key of G

1. What do you know about the relationship between the author and her mother prior to this chapter? What additional information about this relationship do you learn?

2. Music and references to music are used extensively in this chapter. In what capacities?

3. The author is both daughter and therapeutic musician to her mother. Was the dual role harmful and/or beneficial? To whom? Why?

4. Does the author's mother ever consider her daughter a "real" musician? Why or why not?

5. Do you think her mother understands the author's musical gifts? Why or why not?

6. What underlying questions might the author be seeking answers to as she interacts with her mother? Does she receive answers?

Summary questions

1. What new information did you learn about the use of music to promote healing?

2. What themes recur throughout *Musical Morphine*?

3. What characters or events moved you the most? Who, what, and why?

4. What information in *Musical Morphine* made an impression on you? How might it change how you approach illness, aging, dying? As patient? As caregiver? As clinician?

To download a printable copy of these questions, or for links to additional resources, visit www.robingaiser.com/resources.

Acknowledgements

When I read some of the vignettes in this book to the first writers' group I ever attended, the Wednesday group at Barnes & Noble in Asheville, the members sat mesmerized by these accounts of my work. They convinced me that each vignette ought to be expanded into a chapter, and then assembled into a book. I followed their advice and, knowing I had much to learn, enrolled in classes through ClarityWorks with Peggy Tabor Millin. There I began trusting my writing voice and believing I had something worthwhile to say.

These classes were followed by several at UNC Asheville's Great Smokies Writing Program, where Professors Christina Hale and Brian Lee Knopp, and, later, Tina Barr, encouraged my writing with honest critique as well as unsolicited praise. Brian urged me to consider advanced prose class taught by Tommy Hays, Director of the Great Smokies program.

To be admitted to that class I had to commit to a project and submit something I had already written. To my joy, Professor Hayes accepted me into his twelve-person seminar, and *Musical Morphine* became a serious endeavor. Monthly deadlines for eighteen pages of new or newly revised manuscript, oral and written critiques from classmates and Professor Hays, plus weekly reading assignments of short stories and "how-to" books on writing, honed my writing skills and broadened my view of the craft of written expression.

As the book took shape the following generous people contributed their various talents to the developing manuscript. Julie Abbott was my first professional editor. Amy Campbell, Jane Ferguson, Jan Getz, Judith Hoy, Beth Hunt, Laurel Hunt, Sunny Kruger, Carol Lisi, Dwight Martin, Lois McMahon, Martha Mills, Kit Putnam, Nancy West, Sharon West, and the Gunther family, were all keen readers of and listeners to fresh manuscript pages. Another group of reader-reviewers—Donna Marie Castaner, Earl Fowler, Clarie Hicks, Laura Hope-Gill, Kathleen Jablonski, Nick Jacobs, Jeff Jones, Lara McKinnis, Kathy Meacham, Susan Mims, Cam Murchison, and Arlen Rambush—all brought insight to the manuscript from a wide range of expertise.

Laurie McCarriar of Artist Geek created my website, fliers, Thursday email excerpts, photography, and cover design; Misti McCloud, my publicist, oversaw FaceBook and

Twitter, photography, publicity, and events planning and execution. I thank Ben Matcher, Kris Hartrum, and Dave Burr at TalkingBook for audio book recording and editing; Bonnie Cooper of bonniecooperphotography.com for back cover and excerpt photos; and Susan Casler for her wonderful insights and generosity in writing the Foreword to this book.

Last but never least, I'm grateful to my editor and publisher A. D. Reed and his editorial colleague Sarah-Ann Smith at Pisgah Press, whose wisdom, respect, and enthusiasm moved this project forward to places beyond my wildest dreams.

I thank them all for their encouragement, guidance, and support as this book has taken shape and taken wing.

Robin Russell Gaiser

About the Author

Robin Russell Gaiser earned her B.A. in English at The College of William and Mary, where she also sang and played with a folk-rock group, both on campus and in venues in Richmond, Virginia, and Washington, D.C. After graduation she taught writing and literature in Fairfax County, Virginia; then, while raising her family, she gave private lessons in guitar and dulcimer and performed publicly under the auspices of the Fairfax County Council of the Arts. She also sang in classical choirs and joined The Mill Run Dulcimer Band, recording seven albums now included in the Smithsonian collection.

With her children grown, Robin earned an M.A. in psychology from Marymount University and worked as a guidance counselor for eight years. Then, after relocating to upstate N.Y. and becoming caregiver—and bedside musician—for her dying father, she enrolled in a certification program for therapeutic musicians. As a Certified Music Practitioner (CMP), she is trained to provide live, bedside, one-on-one acoustic music to critically and chronically ill, elderly, and dying patients.

After forty-three years in northern Virginia and eight years in upstate New York, Robin and her husband relocated to Asheville, N.C., where she has pursued both her music and her writing careers. Her fiction has appeared in the women's literary journal *Minerva Rising* ("Angels," Dec. 2012) in three anthologies of short stories published by Grateful Steps Publishing (*Drowning Allison & other stories* ("Yellow," 2012), *The Cricket & other stories* ("Doorways," 2014), and *Bits of Sugar & other stories* ("I'll Fly Away," 2016); and in *Writing in Circles: A Celebration of Women's Writing*, published by Sunburst Cabin Press ("Took Out the Tattered," 2014). Her essay "How Music Led Me to Memoir" appeared on the blog, Memoir Writers' Journey, published by Kathy Pooler, in 2014.

Currently pursuing a graduate certificate in Narrative Medicine at Lenoir-Rhyne University's Graduate Center, Robin also volunteers as a musician at homeless shelters, for homebound seniors, and for nonprofit fundraisers. She and her husband are the parents of one daughter and two sons, and grandparents of three.

Also available from Pisgah Press

Barry Burgess
Mombie: The Zombie Mom   illus. by Jake LaGory $16.95

Donna Lisle Burton
Letting Go: Collected Poems 1983-2003 $14.95

Heather A. Houskeeper
A Guide to the Edible and Medicinal Plants of the Finger Lakes Trail $24.00

Michael Hopping
MacTiernan's Bottle $14.95
rhythms on a flaming drum $16.95

C. Robert Jones
I Like It Here! Adventures in the Wild & Wonderful World of Theatre $30.00

LANKY TALES
Vol. I: The Bird Man & other stories   illus. by Jennie Jones Branham $9.00
Vol. II: Billy Red Wing & other stories   illus. by Jane Snyder $9.00
Vol. III: A Good and Faithful Friend & other stories   illus. by Jane Snyder $9.00

Jeff Douglas Messer
Red-state, White-guy Blues $15.95

Patrick O'Sullivan
A Green One for Woody $15.95

A. D. Reed
Reed's Homophones: a comprehensive book of sound-alike words   softcover $10.00
                                           hardcover $16.95

Dave Richards
Swords in Their Hands: George Washington and the Newburgh Conspiracy $24.95
Finalist in the USA Book Awards for History, 2014

Sarah-Ann Smith
Trang Sen: A Novel of Vietnam $19.50

RF Wilson
THE RICK RYDER MYSTERY SERIES
Deadly Dancing $15.95
Killer Weed $14.95

To order:
Pisgah Press, LLC
PO Box 1427, Candler, NC 28715
www.pisgahpress.com